Head and Neck Cancer Clinics

Series editors

Rehan Kazi
Head and Neck Cancer
Manipal University
Manipal, Karnataka, India

Raghav C. Dwivedi
Head and Neck Cancer
Royal Marsden Hospital
London, United Kingdom

Other titles in the series

Clinical Approach to Well-Differentiated Thyroid Cancers
Frederick L. Greene and Andrzej L. Komorowski

Tumours of the Skull Base and Paranasal Sinuses
Ziv Gil and Dan M. Fliss

Controversies in Oral Cancer
K.A. Pathak and Richard W. Nason

HPV and Head and Neck Cancers
Carole Fakhry and Gypsyamber D'Souza

Non-Melanoma Skin Cancer of the Head and Neck
Faruque Riffat, Carsten E. Palme and Michael Veness

K. Alok Pathak · Richard W. Nason
Janice L. Pasieka

Editors

Management of Thyroid Cancer

Special Considerations

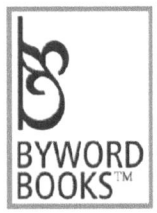

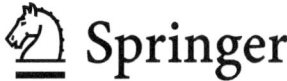

Editors
K. Alok Pathak
University of Manitoba
Manitoba, Canada

Janice L. Pasieka
Head and Neck Surgical Oncology
University of Calgary
Calgary, Canada

Richard W. Nason
Head and Neck Surgical Oncology
Cancer Care Manitoba
Winnipeg, Canada

ISSN 2364-4060   ISSN 2364-4079   (electronic)
Head and Neck Cancer Clinics
ISBN 978-81-322-2433-4   ISBN 978-81-322-2434-1   (eBook)
DOI 10.1007/978-81-322-2434-1

Library of Congress Control Number: 2015943506

Springer New Delhi Heidelberg New York Dordrecht London

Cover illustration by Dan Gibbons DCR(R), PgCert(CT)

Printed on acid-free paper

Springer India Ltd. is part of Springer Science+Business Media (www.springer.com)
Byword Books Private Limited, Delhi, India (www.bywordbooks.in)

This series is dedicated to the research and charity efforts of Cancer Aid and Research Foundation (CARF), Mumbai, India (www.cancerarfoundation.org).

A Note on the Series

Head and neck cancer (HNC) is a major public health challenge. Its management involves a multidisciplinary team approach, which varies depending upon the subtle differences in the location of the tumor, stage and biology of disease, and availability of resources. In the wake of rapidly evolving diagnostic technologies and management techniques, and advances in the basic sciences related to HNC, it is important for both clinicians and basic scientists to be up to date in their knowledge of new diagnostic and management protocols.

This series aims to cover the entire range of HNC-related issues through independent volumes on specific topics. Each volume focuses on a single topic relevant to the current practice of HNC and contains comprehensive chapters written by experts in the field. The reviews in each volume provide vast information on key clinical advances and novel approaches to enable a better understanding of relevant aspects in HNC.

Individual volumes present different perspectives and have the potential to serve as stand-alone reference guides. We believe these volumes will prove useful for the practice of head and neck surgery and oncology. Medical students, residents, clinicians, and general practitioners seeking to develop their knowledge of HNC will benefit from them.

Rehan Kazi
Raghav C. Dwivedi

Preface

Thyroid cancer is the most common malignant endocrine tumor and is the seventh most common cancer seen in Canadians. The incidence of thyroid cancer has been increasing more rapidly than any other cancer in many of the cancer registries from different parts of the world.

Although the majority of thyroid cancers have an indolent biological behavior, different histological types have a diverse clinical behavior. Well-differentiated thyroid cancers have an excellent survival, whereas poorly differentiated and anaplastic thyroid cancers have a very poor outcome. This volume of Head and Neck Cancer Clinics addresses advances, controversies, and state-of-the-art treatment recommendations of various types of thyroid cancers.

This volume on *Management of Thyroid Cancer: Special Considerations* encompasses the molecular risk stratification, management of regional and distant metastatic thyroid cancer, salvage of central compartment recurrence, role of external beam radiation therapy, and posttreatment surveillance of thyroid cancer. Management of medullary and anaplastic thyroid cancer and the evolving role of targeted therapy in thyroid cancer have been discussed in separate chapters. Each chapter is followed by an editorial commentary, which we hope will be enjoyed by the readers.

Winnipeg, MB, Canada   K. Alok Pathak
Winnipeg, MB, Canada   Richard W. Nason
Calgary, AB, Canada   Janice L. Pasieka

Contents

Contributors

Shabirhusain S. Abadin Department of Surgical Oncology, The University of Texas MD Anderson Cancer Center, Houston, TX, USA

Naifa L. Busaidy Department of Endocrine Neoplasia and Hormonal Disorders, The University of Texas MD Anderson Cancer Center, Houston, TX, USA

Laura Chin-Lenn Section of General Surgery and Surgical Oncology, University of Calgary, Calgary, AB, Canada

Sylvie Galindo Department of Surgery, St. Paul's Hospital & University of British Columbia, Vancouver, BC, Canada

Adrian Harvey Department of Surgery, Faculty of Medicine, University of Calgary, Calgary, AB, Canada

Rehan Kazi Manipal University, Manipal, Karnataka, India

Todd P.W. McMullen Division of Surgical Oncology, University of Alberta, Edmonton, AB, Canada

Richard W. Nason Head and Neck Surgical Oncology, CancerCare Manitoba, Winnipeg, MB, Canada

Vicky M. Parkins Division of Endocrinology and Metabolism, Department of Medicine, University of Calgary and Alberta Health Services, Calgary, AB, Canada

Janice L. Pasieka Section of General Surgery and Surgical Oncology, University of Calgary, Calgary, AB, Canada

J.D. Pasternak Division of General Surgery, Toronto General Hospital, University Health Network, Toronto, ON, Canada

K. Alok Pathak Head and Neck Surgical Oncology, CancerCare Manitoba, University of Manitoba, Winnipeg, MB, Canada

Nancy D. Perrier Department of Surgical Oncology, The University of Texas MD Anderson Cancer Center, Houston, TX, USA

Harvey Quon Radiation Oncology, CancerCare Manitoba, Winnipeg, MB, Canada

L.E. Rotstein Division of General Surgery, Toronto General Hospital, University Health Network, Toronto, ON, Canada

Erik S. Venos Division of Endocrinology and Metabolism, Department of Medicine, University of Calgary and Alberta Health Services, Calgary, AB, Canada

David C. Williams Division of General Surgery, University of Alberta, Edmonton, AB, Canada

Sam M. Wiseman Department of Surgery, St. Paul's Hospital & University of British Columbia, Vancouver, BC, Canada

Abbreviations

3DCRT	3-Dimensional conformal radiotherapy
AGES	Age, grade, extent, size
AJCC	American Joint Committee on Cancer
AMES	Age, metastasis, extent, size
AN	Accessory nerve
ATA	American Thyroid Association
ATC	Anaplastic thyroid cancer/carcinoma
ATP	Adenosine triphosphate
BTA	British Thyroid Association
CCA	Common carotid artery
CCH	C-cell hyperplasia
CEA	Carcino-embryonic antigen
cN0	Clinically negative node
CNLND	Central neck lymph node dissection
CSS	Cause-specific survival
CT	Computed tomography
CTV	Clinical target volume
DTC	Differentiated thyroid cancer/carcinoma
EBRT	External beam radiotherapy
EGFR	Endothelial-derived growth factor receptor
EMT	Epithelial-to-mesenchymal transition
EORTC	European Organization for Research and Treatment of Cancer
FDA	US Food and Drug Administration
FDG-PET	Fludeoxyglucose positron emission tomography
FMTC	Familial medullary thyroid cancer
FNA	Fine-needle aspiration
FNAB	Fine-needle aspiration biopsy
FTC	Follicular thyroid cancer/carcinoma
HCC	Hürthle cell carcinoma
HNC	Head and neck cancer/carcinoma
IMRT	Intensity-modulated radiotherapy
IONM	Intraoperative nerve monitoring
LN	Lymph node
MACIS	Metastasis, age, completeness of resection, invasion, size (score)

MAPK	Mitogen-activated protein kinase
MEN	Multiple endocrine neoplasia
MEN2	Multiple endocrine neoplasia type 2
MRI	Magnetic resonance imaging
MTC	Medullary thyroid cancer/carcinoma
NCCN	National Comprehensive Cancer Network
NPV	Negative predictive value
NTRK	Neurotrophic tyrosine receptor kinase
pCLND	Prophylactic central neck dissection
PDGFR	Platelet-derived growth factor receptor
PET	Positron emission tomography
PFS	Progression-free survival
PPV	Positive predictive value
PR	Partial response
PTC	Papillary thyroid cancer/carcinoma
PTH	Parathyroid hormone
RAI	Radioactive iodine
RAS	Rat sarcoma oncogene
RCC	Renal cell carcinoma
RECIST	Response evaluation criteria in solid tumors
RET	Rearranged during transformation
RFA	Radiofrequency ablation
rhTSH	Recombinant human thyroid-stimulating hormone
RLN	Recurrent laryngeal nerve
Rt RLN	Right recurrent laryngeal nerve
RTK	Receptor tyrosine kinase
SCC	Squamous cell carcinoma
SCM	Sternocleidomastoid muscle
SD	Stable disease
SEER	Surveillance, Epidemiology and End Results (database)
SLNB	Sentinel lymph node biopsy
STAT3	Signal transducers and activators of transcription-3
SUV	Standard uptake value
Tg	Thyroglobulin
TGF-β	Transforming growth factor beta
THW	Thyroid hormone withdrawal
TK	Tyrosine kinase
TKI	Tyrosine kinase inhibitor
TSH	Thyroid-stimulating hormone
VEGF	Vascular endothelial growth factor
VEGFR	Vascular endothelial growth factor receptor
WDTC	Well-differentiated thyroid cancer/carcinoma

Molecular Risk Stratification of Well-Differentiated Thyroid Cancer

Todd P.W. McMullen and David C. Williams

The Burden of Disease and Current Limitations of Thyroid Cytopathology

Papillary and follicular variants comprise the majority (>90 %) of thyroid carcinomas [1]. The worldwide incidence of WDTC is increasing significantly; age-adjusted rates in North America and Europe are now over twice that documented in 1990 [2, 3]. Increased use of ultrasound in thyroid assessments for nodular disease is cited as an important factor driving the increased incidence of thyroid cancer [2, 4]. Nearly 50 % of nodules identified by ultrasound are in patients lacking risk factors or clinical signs and symptoms of nodular disease. It is reasonable to quote the expected prevalence of nodular disease in ≤25 % of the population [5, 6]. Investigation of thyroid neoplasms will continue to pose a significant clinical and financial burden to the healthcare system.

The diagnostic workhorse employed by physicians to detect thyroid malignancy is FNAB [6–8]. This quick and easy test to sample cells within the thyroid neoplasm is considered the most important tool in assessing patients for thyroid cancer. Empirical evidence supporting the use of fine-needle aspiration (FNA) cytology in the risk stratification of malignancy in thyroid nodules has been well established through multiple randomized trials [9–12]. Historically, when a sufficient number of cells were obtained by FNAB, results were divided into three categories: indeterminate, benign or malignant. It is commonly quoted that ≤1 in 4 patients may have an indeterminate

T.P.W. McMullen (✉)
Division of Surgical Oncology, University of Alberta, Edmonton, AB, Canada
e-mail: Todd.Mcmullen@albertahealthservices.ca

D.C. Williams
Division of General Surgery, University of Alberta, Edmonton, AB, Canada
e-mail: dcw@ualberta.ca

© K. Alok Pathak, Richard W. Nason, Janice L. Pasieka, Rehan Kazi,
Raghav C. Dwivedi 2015
Springer India/Byword Books
K.A. Pathak et al. (eds.), *Management of Thyroid Cancer: Special Considerations*,
Head and Neck Cancer Clinics, DOI 10.1007/978-81-322-2434-1_1

result [10]. The Bethesda system for reporting thyroid cytopathology was generated to clarify communication between pathologists and physicians and for reliable comparison of data obtained at different sites [10]. The positive predictive value of FNAB has decreased the number of diagnostic procedures for benign disease, with >70 % of resected specimens revealing malignancy [12]. This represents a substantial improvement over the pre-FNAB period, which relied primarily on clinical assessments. Ultrasound-guided FNAB and improved cytology reporting have increased diagnostic accuracy and decreased unnecessary surgery but there are limits to further improvements. Most of the uncertainty in thyroid nodule cytopathology involves follicular lesions of undetermined significance and follicular neoplasms with and without atypia. The risk of malignancy in these groups of 'indeterminate' lesions varies between 5 and 30 % in the refined Bethesda criteria [10]. In the next step of the diagnostic paradigm, i.e. surgery, only 20 % of patients turn out to have malignancy; in other words, 4 of 5 patients would not have required diagnostic surgery if more accurate testing was available [11]. The diagnostic certainty with FNAB, while better with 75–80 % of cases defined as suspicious for malignancy, still means that nearly 1 in 4 patients will have surgery for benign disease [12]. In addition to the problem with indeterminate specimens, it is possible that FNAB might miss thyroid cancers altogether. Even in high-volume centres with specialized endocrine pathologists, when used to classify thyroid nodules FNAB provides an accurate diagnosis in only 70 % of all cases in a large meta-analysis [13]. Sampling error could also be an important factor. A recent study quoted the rate of missed cancers, the false-negative rate, at approximately one in three palpable nodules, but these findings have been disputed by other studies [14, 15]. It is clear that the accuracy of FNAB is limited. Extremes of size, nodules of <5 mm or >4 cm, or where autoimmune disease coexists, may make it difficult to accurately obtain a representative tumour biopsy [14, 15].

The shortcomings of FNAB are not limited to differentiating benign from malignant disease. Patients diagnosed with WDTC will require a total thyroidectomy, possibly followed by radioactive iodine treatment to remove small deposits of residual thyroid or metastatic tumour [8]. Lymphatic metastases are associated with increased risk of locoregional recurrence, which significantly impairs quality of life and is linked to a poorer prognosis in patients >45 years of age [16–24]. Currently, there are no histological or genetic markers accepted as predictors of lymphatic disease. Imaging techniques, including high-resolution ultrasound, are also relatively insensitive to nodal metastases [25, 26]. Thus, the only way to rule out lymphatic metastases is to prophylactically remove the nodes within the central neck (level VI lymph node dissection) [27]. The routine use of central compartment node dissections is associated with increased risk to the recurrent laryngeal nerve and a multifold increase in the risk of hypoparathyroidism and the need for the patient to require lifelong calcium supplementation [28, 29]. Consequently, surgeons are faced with the decision to risk undertreating a patient if they do not extirpate level VI lymph nodes, or overtreating with a more complete removal of nodes with a thyroidectomy, possibly causing lifelong complications. Ideally, testing of tumour FNAB samples for biomarkers of aggressive behaviour and a propensity for lymphatic spread would allow surgeons to more accurately identify those patients needing more extensive level VI neck dissections.

It is clear that cytopathological assessment could be improved by adjunct testing to stratify benign and malignant disease and minimize the need for diagnostic surgery. Adjunct tests may also assist surgeons in properly selecting thyroid carcinoma patients with aggressive tumours for more extensive lymph node dissections while also minimizing procedures and risk for those patients with indolent tumours. The need for this test to evolve is urgent in an era of increasing incidence of this disease and financial restraints on healthcare systems.

Oncogenesis in WDTC

Opportunities for novel diagnostic tools come directly from studies examining how changes in gene and protein expression translate into the unique thyroid cancer phenotypes [30–34]. Thyroid cancer develops through a combination of genetic and epigenetic changes. Changes in gene expression through chromosomal rearrangements and point mutations are well known to drive thyroid oncogenesis, as can be observed by signature changes in thyroid cancer morphology and clinical behaviour. Of relevance to this chapter, it is understood that four mutually exclusive genetic lesions account for >90 % of cases of papillary thyroid carcinoma (PTC): fusion oncoproteins rearranged in transformation/PTC (RET/PTC) or neurotrophic tyrosine receptor kinase (NTRK) and activating mutations of the BRAF or rat sarcoma oncogene (RAS) genes [30–34]. The RET proto-oncogene and NTRK are both tyrosine kinase genes that can be activated by chromosomal rearrangement with other genes of unrelated function. The known number of RET/PTC arrangements is in excess of 16 but RET/PTC1 and RET/PTC3 are by far the ones most commonly found in papillary carcinomas [35–39]. Cellular transformation via RET/PTC mutations most commonly activate the RAS/RAF/MEK/MAPK pathway [35, 37, 40, 41]. Whereas the MAPK pathway is considered a key element in the transformation for thyroid cancer, it is clear that the signal transducers and activators of transcription-3 (STAT3) pathway, a known oncogenic factor, is also activated in RET/PTC rearrangements [42–44]. RET/PTC mutations typically occur at a younger age, have a classic histopathology and commonly spread to lymph nodes [30, 33]. It is important to note that other mutations or epigenetic changes are required to complete the neoplastic process, as RET/PTC transgenic mice have been shown to have a considerable lag time before tumours form. [45] BRAF, an isoform of a class of serine-threonine kinases, is a member of the RAF/MEK/MAPK signalling pathway that regulates a number of important cellular processes, such as proliferation and cell-cycle progression. The V600E mutation in BRAF is an important and well conserved mutation in PTC that generates a high level of MAP kinase activity [30–33, 46, 47]. This mutation occurs as an initiating event; however, its upregulation of the RAS/RAF/MEK/MAPK pathway is not thought sufficient to transform thyroid cells, as was found previously for RET/ PTC translocations [31, 48]. It is postulated that the BRAF mutation causes secondary genetic events which activate other pathways, including STAT3, PI3K/Akt and mTOR, allowing thyroid tumour progression [49, 50]. Tumours with the BRAF gene mutation typically exhibit aggressive characteristics, including extrathyroidal extension, advanced stage at diagnosis and lymph node metastases [30, 33, 51]. RAS genes encode membrane G-proteins that play a role in signal transduction. Mutations in RAS can activate the number of pathways, including the RAS/RAF/MEK/MAPK pathway, as well as the PI3K/Akt and STAT3 pathways [30, 31, 49, 50]. The point mutations in RAS genes occur in ~10 % of papillary thyroid tumours and typically lead to tumours resembling more follicular variant histology with a low rate of lymph node metastases [31]. PAX8/PPARg is another fusion protein that drives oncogenesis but it is most commonly associated with follicular thyroid carcinoma (FTC), as opposed to PTC. It can be found in benign tumours as well, and relatively little is known regarding downstream changes in the signalling activity that lead to malignant transformation of thyroid nodules [30].

The progression of thyroid carcinoma to metastases has also recently been linked to the epithelial-to-mesenchymal transition (EMT), a process involving loss of cell-cell contacts and remodelling of the cytoskeleton [52, 53]. Transforming growth factor beta (TGF-β) has also been shown to induce the EMT transition in a mouse model of thyroid cancer [53]. Growth factor receptors, such as EGFR and PDGFR, are also known to activate multiple pathways (e.g. PI3K/Akt and MAPK/ERK) to induce cell migration, invasion, and angiogenesis consistent with the EMT phenotype in many other tumour types, and thus may also play a role in thyroid carcinoma [54]. WDTC have a significant propensity for nodal metastases and much may be learned from the examination of growth factor signalling and activation pathways linked to EMT, such as PI3K/Akt [51].

Oncogenesis in thyroid follicular cells may also be driven through epigenetic changes as well as through variations in microRNA (miRNA) expression [55]. miRNA expression profiles have been completed on malignant and benign thyroid nodules identifying possible failed regulators of gene expression that contribute to the progression of thyroid cancer, such as miR-221. Other genetic regulatory mechanisms, including methylation, may also contribute to different thyroid carcinoma phenotypes. For example, altered methylation of the promoter site for metalloproteinase genes and subsequent changes in protein expression, may alter the ability of the cells to migrate and present as nodal or distant disease [56].

Molecular Diagnostics and Innovations in Thyroid Cancer Diagnostics

The effort to identify diagnostic molecular markers in thyroid cancer spans 15 years and includes mutational analysis, immunohistochemical studies of changes in protein expression, as well as changes in mRNA and miRNA levels.

Current Status of Gene Testing in Tumour Specimens

RET/PTC

Attempts to stratify malignant and benign thyroid nodules began with examination of the common RET/PTC, BRAF and other mutations that are well defined in differentiated thyroid cancer. Recent reports comment that molecular testing for somatic mutations represents a promising diagnostic approach [51]. To avoid limitations in tissue sampling and access, the first studies examined fresh and paraffin-embedded tumour specimens in an attempt to correlate the presence of these mutations with carcinoma and poor patient outcomes [51]. The RET/PTC translocation was one of the first genes recognized as a marker for carcinogenesis in thyrocytes and has been reviewed extensively [51, 57, 58]. A significant effort was made to demonstrate the utility of genetic testing for this translocation as a means to identifying malignant lesions, particularly when pathologists had labelled the specimens as having indeterminate risk for malignancy [51, 57]. However, it is now clear that RET/PTC rearrangements are found in both carcinomas and benign neoplasms. [58] It has also been observed that not all of the cells within a given tumour may demonstrate RET/PTC rearrangements, and what was previously thought to represent an early event in tumourigenesis is, in fact, a subclone in only a portion of the cells within the tumour [57, 58]. Marotta et al., in a thorough review, revealed that the subcloned occurrence of RET/PTC translocations may account for the dramatic variations in prevalence shown in different studies [57]. Consequently, the clinical utility of RET/PTC testing as a means to differentiating malignant and benign lesions from indeterminate cytopathology is limited.

BRAF

Constitutive activation of the MAP kinase pathway is associated strongly with WDTC and this has been the basis for studies into the BRAF mutation and its role in patient outcomes. Two meta-analyses of the V600E BRAF mutation and the clinico-pathological features of thyroid cancer demonstrated that the average prevalence rate was nearly 50 % of all PTC cases in a compilation of over 26 studies that spanned the globe [59, 60].' It is also clear that cases of WDTC with this mutation were twice as likely to exhibit extrathyroidal extension as well as advanced TNM stage. Lymph node metastases were also 1.5 times more likely in patients with the BRAF mutation. It is worth noting that in a review by Kim et al., the authors searched only for the V600E variant and included patients only with tumours of >2 cm, which means that patients with smaller tumours were underrepresented in this systematic review [59]. Other investigators have shown that even in tumours of <2 cm, the presence of BRAF is associated with more advanced disease [61]. Overall, >2,000 patients were included in these meta-analyses and it is clear that BRAF has an important role in thyroid oncogenesis that is relevant for treatment planning.

RAS

Mutations of the RAS gene, in three variants H-, N- and K-, have also been examined with respect to tumour morphology and patient outcome [30, 51, 62]. These mutations are spread broadly across both papillary and FTCs. RAS mutations activate both the MAPK and PI3K/Akt pathways. Tumours with the RAS mutation demonstrate follicular morphology associated with follicular variants of PTC [63]. Benign thyroid nodules also have a significant incidence of RAS mutations, in some cases ≤40 % of follicular adenomas [64, 65]. RAS mutations, when combined with other transforming factors, may also drive dedifferentiation. For example, in cases with combined BRAF and RAS mutations, the tumours are associated with distant metastases and poor outcomes [66, 67].

PAX8/PPARg

Fewer studies have investigated the role of the PAX8/PPARg gene fusion in predicting malignancy or the morphology of thyroid tumours and patient outcomes [32, 34, 48]. It is clear that this protein is more frequent in FTCs but benign tumours also exhibit this gene rearrangement. In one study examining tumour morphology and staging, this fusion protein was associated with tumours more commonly found in women and with more differentiated tumours, as well as with favourable prognosis through decreased incidence of metastatic disease [68].

Current Status of Gene Testing in FNAB Specimens

Advances in ultrasound and standardization of FNAB reporting (using the Bethesda criteria) have minimized non-diagnostic and indeterminate specimens. However, up to one in four attempts fail to make a definitive diagnosis. Ultrasound is increasingly sensitive and more readily available and thus the number of nodules requiring biopsies is likely to continue to increase in the coming years. This further illustrates the need for molecular biomarkers to utilize the clinicopathological correlations associated with unique gene mutations (e.g. BRAF) to address the limits of cytopathology in predicting malignancy.

Single-Gene Studies

The important role of the BRAF gene in thyroid oncogenesis is reflected in the number of studies that have used this gene to predict malignancy in FNAB specimens. Mehta et al. (2012) compiled a mix of prospective trials and retrospective cohorts examining the association of the BRAF mutation with differentiated thyroid cancer in >2,000 patients [69]. One of the essential clinical points to be generated is that the false-positive rate is very low when examining malignant tumours for the presence of the V600E BRAF mutation. The high specificity of the BRAF testing was confirmed in a separate meta-analysis [70]. A detailed examination of the BRAF mutation in surgically resected specimens indicates that the V600E mutation is associated with classic variants of PTC, whereas the K601E mutation is associated with the follicular variant of PTC and is more likely to be seen in FNA specimens characterized as follicular lesions of unknown significance [71]. Some authors have stated that the presence of a BRAF mutation in an indeterminate FNA specimen could designate that nodule as PTC by convention [69]. However, the application of the BRAF test to almost 500 indeterminate lesions surgically removed and pathologically defined by Filicori et al. revealed that mutation analysis may only identify one-third of the malignancies within this group of specimens [72]. Even when the mutation analysis was negative in an FNAB specimen classified as indeterminate, the authors quote an overall risk of malignancy of nearly one in four. Atypia was an important predictor of risk regardless of mutation status [72]. Thus, many indeterminate nodules on final pathology represent carcinomas that lack the BRAF mutation. Similar to that found with BRAF mutations, the presence of RET/PTC fusion transcripts in indeterminate specimens is highly specific for differentiated thyroid carcinomas [70]. However, as reviewed by Ferraz et al., once again a single-gene analysis for the RET/PTC gene lacks sensitivity; therefore, even in the presence of a negative test, the risk of cancer may be two or three times that of the general population, prompting surgical intervention for definitive diagnosis [70]. Comparatively little data exist on gene testing of FNAB specimens for RAS mutations and PAX8/ PPARg rearrangements as a means to identify malignancy. In both cases mutations can be detected in both benign and malignant lesions, thereby limiting their accuracy [70, 73].

Mutational Analysis Using Gene Panels

To overcome the limits of individual gene analysis, a handful of studies have examined multiple markers in FNAB specimens as a means to improving the sensitivity of molecular diagnostics. A recent trial of over 1,000 patients, of whom nearly 500 had surgery, the risk of malignancy for cases defined as: (i) atypia of undetermined significance/follicular lesion of undetermined significance, (ii) follicular neoplasm or (iii) suspicious for malignancy was (i) 88 %, (ii) 87 %, and (iii) 95 %, respectively, in the presence of any mutation [71]. The RAS mutations comprised nearly 75 % of all the mutations found, followed by BRAF and a few RET/PTC and PPAR gamma mutations. However, even in tumours with none of the common mutations, a significant risk remains of cancer when the histopathology is defined as indeterminate [71]. Generally, similar results have been reported by other authors using a combination of the four major mutations associated with differentiated thyroid cancer [51, 62, 69–75]. It is clear that gene panels that include some combination of BRAF, RET/PTC, RAS and PAX8/PPARg mutations are >90 % specific but the sensitivity varies significantly between 38 % and 80 % in the different studies [70]. For example, in a prospective trial by Mathur et al. (2010) in which all the common somatic mutations outlined above were examined for 400 nodules in 341 patients, the authors revealed a 10 % rate of somatic mutations even in benign nodules [9].

Discriminating Benign Nodular Disease and Thyroid Cancer Using Gene Expression Arrays

Gene expression profiles have also been utilized to identify possible diagnostic bio-markers that can distinguish benign from malignant thyroid neoplasms in FNAB specimens. In a large meta-analysis by Griffith et al., the authors examined 21 early studies using a gene ranking system to outline significant up- or down-regulation of genes associated with PTC and FTC tumours [76]. In this analysis, a series of 12 genes could distinguish between benign and malignant thyroid disease [76]. Not all of the gene products generated by the array are known and only a handful were vali-dated by both qRT-PCR and immunohistochemistry. Refinements on these earlier studies using surgically removed specimens have led to attempts to use gene expres-sion levels of selected markers to distinguish between benign and malignant lesions on FNAB specimens [51, 77–80]. Differentially expressed genes, including ANGPT2, ARG2, EGFR, hTERT, TFF3, TIMP1 and TMPRSS4, have been used in different studies to classify benign from malignant lesions. Further refinements in gene testing, as shown in studies by Prasad et al., have led to a three-gene model that can distinguish benign and malignant Amours from FNA specimens classified as indeterminate with a sensitivity of ~80 % and virtually 100 % specificity [81]. In 2012, gene array technology for discriminating benign and malignant Amours from indeterminate FNAB specimens became commercially accessible to physicians and patients [82]. For example, Walsh et al. examined the clinical application of a gene expression classifier kit to demonstrate that the methods of gene analysis were robust and reproducible under clinical testing conditions [83]. A recent prospective, multicentre trial involving nearly 5,000 FNAB specimens demonstrated that this technology could discern benign from malignant specimens, previously classified as indeterminate by histopathology, with >90 % sensitivity [84]. The negative pre-dictive values were ≥90 % for follicular neoplasms. [84] As a result, the authors report that the use of this tool could allow clinicians to take a more conservative approach with respect to indeterminate lesions and thereby minimize diagnostic surgery.

Other Testing Platforms and Strategies Under Evaluation

Protein Biomarkers

Immunohistochemistry has been applied for a number of years to thyroid specimens to generate prognostic and diagnostic tools. Of the many studies that have examined the expression of individual proteins and their association with malignancy in thy-roid cancer, galectin-3, HBME-1, and CK-19 stand out as the proteins most commonly cited [85]. Galectin-3, which has been studied prospectively and given its high specificity for staining malignant Amours, was demonstrated as a useful adjunct to the cytological assessment of thyroid nodules [85]. However, as reviewed by Chiu et al. (2010), the reported accuracy varies beleen studies, which may explain why it has not been adopted in general [85]. A comparison of studies is also difficult because of the use of different cut-offs for determining negative and positive immunohistochemical staining, lack of standardization for describing staining patterns, and differences in protocol for antibody staining [86]. For HMBE-1 and CK-19, the sensitivity and specificity again vary beleen different studies and a significant portion of benign nodules exhibit strong staining [85, 87]. Of a host of other proteins, some of which are reviewed by Rodrigues et al. (2012), it is clear that many markers are either sensitive or specific but neither have the required accuracy to be suitable for clinical testing [62]. Much work has been done on surgical specimens which has not been tested for antibody sensitivity, binding and scoring using cytological aspirates that present novel challenges to immunocytochemical analysis, given the small amount of material. However, access to additional tissue can be addressed with the use of larger bore needles, as has been shown for galectin-3 [88].

mRNA

Control of mRNA translation and degradation by miRNA represents a level of gene regulation in addition to gene transcription that has a significant impact on tumourigenesis [89]. Differentiation of benign and malignant thyroid nodules has been completed on surgical specimens with miRNA-7, -146, -221 that have a strong association with malignancy [90, 91]. Profiling also identifies specific signatures for miRNA expression in benign, well-differentiated and anaplastic thyroid cancers [90–92]. Until recently, few studies have evaluated the utility of miRNA analysis using FNAB to guide therapy [93–95]. Kitano et al. (2012) examined the expression of four miRNAs in benign and malignant biopsy specimens to reveal that miRNA-7 was the single best predictor of malignancy with a high sensitivity (100 %), but low (<30 %) specificity [90]. A series of four miRNAs (miRNA-100, -125b, -138, -768-3p) showed significant differences in expression with respect to benign and malignant thyroid neoplasms. [91] As with proteins and DNA-based studies, it appears that individual miRNAs do not provide sufficient accuracy, but combining markers does increase the accuracy to ~80 % overall [93–95]. Analysis of FNAB specimens for miRNA signatures thus represent another option for classifying indeterminate lesions, but this work is in its early stages.

Conclusion and Future Directions

DNA, RNA and protein sampling have been trialled as methods to identify biomarkers suitable for predicting malignancy in thyroid neoplasms. The increasing burden of thyroid nodular disease will continue to drive molecular diagnostics. Any test of clinical utility will have to meet the demands of FNAB sampling that provides limited cell numbers, requires fixatives or air drying, and limits the quality and quantity of protein, RNA and DNA for expression analysis. Consequently, few tools have the required simplicity, reproducibility or accuracy to become widely accepted as an adjunct to cytological analysis of thyroid aspirates. Despite these challenges the number of published articles promoting molecular diagnostics increases every year. Evidence of progress is illustrated by the work of Alexander et al. (2012) in which gene expression profiling can discriminate benign from malignant disease with a high degree of accuracy when applied to specimens in which cytology was indeterminate [84]. Given recent advances and the appearance of multiple commercial interests, physicians may soon be able to routinely combine gene expression and mutation analysis with cytopathology to predict malignancy in thyroid neoplasms.

Commentary

K. Alok Pathak

The diagnosis of well-differentiated thyroid cancer (WDTC) is often made by fine-needle aspiration biopsy (FNAB); however, differentiating benign and malignant follicular neoplasms remains a challenge that often requires a diagnostic hemithyroidectomy or lobectomy. Encouraging results have been obtained by improving the diagnostic potential of aspiration biopsies through molecular diagnostics, such as gene expression, protein and miRNA profiling. Future developments to define distinct benign and malignant signatures in thyroid neoplasms are likely to include immunocytochemical markers combined with mutation analysis and large-scale genetic sequencing.

In this chapter, Doctors McMullen and Williams discuss the limitations of conventional cytology and the possible diagnostic role of molecular signatures that have been derived from the studies examining how changes in gene and protein expression translate into the unique thyroid cancer phenotypes. In the near future, physicians may be able to routinely combine gene expression and mutation analysis with cytopathology to predict malignancy in thyroid neoplasms. FNAB sampling will continue to remain a challenge, as it provides a limited number of cells and requires fixatives or air drying, which restricts the quality and quantity of protein, RNA and DNA for expression analysis. Furthermore, it does not fulfil the criteria of simplicity, reproducibility and accuracy, for it to become accepted widely as an adjunct to routine cytological analysis for the accuracy of thyroid aspirates.

References

1. Kent WD, Hall SF, Isotalo PA, et al. Increased incidence of differentiated thyroid carcinoma and detection of subclinical disease. CMAJ. 2007;177:1357–61.
2. Li N, Du X, Reitzel L, et al. Impact of enhanced detection on the increase in thyroid cancer incidence in the US: review of incidence trends by socioeconomic status within the surveillance, epidemiology, and end results registry, 1980–2008. Thyroid. 2013;23:103–10.

3. Agate L, Lorusso L, Elisei R. New and old knowledge on differentiated thyroid cancer epidemiology and risk factors. J Endocrinol Invest. 2012;35(6 Suppl):3–9.
4. Ezzat S, Sarti DA, Cain DR, et al. Thyroid incidentalomas. Prevalence by palpation and ultrasonography. Arch Intern Med. 1994;154:1838–40.
5. Yuen AP, Ho AC, Wong BY. Ultrasonographic screening for occult thyroid cancer. Head Neck. 2011;33:453–7.
6. Gharib H, Goellner JR. Fine-needle aspiration biopsy of the thyroid: an appraisal. Ann Intern Med. 1993;118:282–9.
7. Berker D, Aydin Y, Ustun I, et al. The value of fine-needle aspiration biopsy in subcentimeter thyroid nodules. Thyroid. 2008;18:603–8.
8. The American Thyroid Association (ATA) guidelines taskforce on thyroid nodules and differentiated thyroid cancer, Cooper DS, Doherty GM, Haugen BR, et al. Revised American Thyroid Association management guidelines for patients with thyroid nodules and differentiated thyroid cancer. Thyroid. 2009;19:1167–214.
9. Mathur A, Weng J, Moses W, et al. A prospective study evaluating the accuracy of using combined clinical factors and candidate diagnostic markers to refine the accuracy of thyroid fine needle aspiration biopsy. Surgery. 2010;148:1170–6; discussion 1176–7.
10. Wang CC, Friedman L, Kennedy GC, et al. A large multicenter correlation study of thyroid nodule cytopathology and histopathology. Thyroid. 2011;21:243–51.
11. Lewis CM, Chang KP, Pitman M, et al. Thyroid fine-needle aspiration biopsy: variability in reporting. Thyroid. 2009;19:717–23.
12. Layfield LJ, Cibas ES, Baloch Z. Thyroid fine needle aspiration cytology: a review of the National Cancer Institute state of the science symposium. Cytopathology. 2010;21:75–85.
13. Bongiovanni M, Spitale A, Faquin WC, et al. The Bethesda system for reporting thyroid cytopathology: a meta-analysis. Acta Cytol. 2012;56:333–9.
14. Tee YY, Lowe AJ, Brand CA, et al. Fine-needle aspiration may miss a third of all malignancy in palpable thyroid nodules: a comprehensive literature review. Ann Surg. 2007;246:714–20.
15. Roh MH, Jo VY, Stelow EB, et al. The predictive value of the fine-needle aspiration diagnosis 'suspicious for a follicular neoplasm, hurthle cell type' in patients with hashimoto thyroiditis. Am J Clin Pathol. 2011;135:139–45.
16. Tissell LE. Role of lymphadenectomy in the treatment of differentiated thyroid carcinomas. Br J Surg. 1998;85:1025–6.
17. Rotstein L. The role of lymphadenectomy in the management of papillary carcinoma of the thyroid. J Surg Oncol. 2009;99:186–8.
18. Wada N, Duh QY, Sugino K, et al. Lymph node metastasis from 259 papillary thyroid microcarcinomas: frequency, pattern of occurrence and recurrence, and optimal strategy for neck dissection. Ann Surg. 2003;237:399–407.
19. Harwood J, Clark OH, Dunphy JE. Significance of lymph node metastasis in differentiated thyroid cancer. Am J Surg. 1978;136:107–12.
20. Mazzaferri EL, Young L. Papillary thyroid carcinoma: a 10 year follow-up report of the impact of therapy in 576 patients. Am J Med. 1981;70:511–8.
21. Low TH, Delbridge L, Sidhu S, et al. Lymph node status influences follow-up thyroglobulin levels in papillary thyroid cancer. Ann Surg Oncol. 2008;15:2827–32.
22. Verburg FA, Mäder U, Tanase K, et al. Life expectancy is reduced in differentiated thyroid cancer patients ≥45 years old with extensive local tumor invasion, lateral lymph node, or distant metastases at diagnosis and normal in all other DTC patients. J Clin Endocrinol Metab. 2013;98:172–80.
23. Smith VA, Sessions RB, Lentsch EJ. Cervical lymph node metastasis and papillary thyroid carcinoma: does the compartment involved affect survival? Experience from the SEER database. J Surg Oncol. 2012;106:357–62.
24. Lundgren CI, Hall P, Dickman PW, et al. Clinically significant prognostic factors for differentiated thyroid carcinoma: a population-based, nested case–control study. Cancer. 2006;106:524–31.
25. Choi JS, Chung WY, Kwak JY, et al. Staging of papillary thyroid carcinoma with ultrasonography: performance in a large series. Ann Surg Oncol. 2011;18:3572–8.

26. Ito Y, Amino N, Miyauchi A. Thyroid ultrasonography. World J Surg. 2010;34:1171–80.
27. Sywak M, Cornford L, Roach P, et al. Routine ipsilateral level VI lymphadenectomy reduces postoperative thyroglobulin levels in papillary thyroid cancer. Surgery. 2006;140:1000–5; discussion 1005–7.
28. White ML, Doherty GM. Level VI lymph node dissection for papillary thyroid cancer. Minerva Chir. 2007;62:383–93.
29. Sakorafas GH, Sampanis D, Safioleas M. Cervical lymph node dissection in papillary thyroid cancer: current trends, persisting controversies, and unclarified uncertainties. Surg Oncol. 2010;19:e57–70.
30. Nikiforov YE. Thyroid carcinoma: molecular pathways and therapeutic targets. Mod Pathol. 2008;21:S37–43.
31. Riesco-Eizaguirrea G, Santisteban P. Molecular biology of thyroid cancer initiation. Clin Transl Oncol. 2007;9:686–93.
32. Taccaliti A, Boscaro M. Genetic mutations in thyroid carcinoma. Minerva Endocrinol. 2009;34:11–28.
33. Riesco-Eizaguirre G, Santisteban P. New insights in thyroid follicular cell biology and its impact in thyroid cancer therapy. Endocr Relat Cancer. 2007;14:957–77.
34. DeLellis RA. Pathology and genetics of thyroid carcinoma. J Surg Oncol. 2006;94:662–9.
35. Richardson DS, Gujral TS, Peng S, et al. Transcript level modulates the inherent oncogenicity of RET/PTC oncoproteins. Cancer Res. 2009;69:4861–9.
36. Shibru D, Chung KW, Kebebew E. Recent developments in the clinical application of thyroid cancer biomarkers. Curr Opin Oncol. 2008;20:13–8.
37. Cassinelli G, Favini E, Degl'Innocenti D, et al. RET/PTC1-driven neoplastic transformation and proinvasive phenotype of human thyrocytes involve met induction and beta-catenin nuclear translocation. Neoplasia. 2009;11:10–21.
38. Greco A, Miranda C, Pierotti MA. Rearrangements of NTRK1 gene in papillary thyroid carcinoma. Mol Cell Endocrinol. 2010;321:44–9.
39. Ciampi R, Nikiforov YE. RET/PTC rearrangements and BRAF mutations in thyroid tumorigenesis. Endocrinology. 2007;148:936–41.
40. Buckwalter TL, Venkateswaran A, Lavender M, et al. The roles of phosphotyrosines-294, -404, and -451 in RET/PTC1-induced thyroid tumor formation. Oncogene. 2002;21:8166–72.
41. Knauf JA, Kuroda H, Basu S, et al. RET/PTC induced dedifferentiation of thyroid cells is mediated through Y1062 signaling through SHC-RAS-MAP kinase. Oncogene. 2003;22:4406–12.
42. Hwang JH, Kim DW, Suh JM, et al. Activation of signal transducer and activator of transcription 3 by oncogenic RET/PTC (rearranged in transformation/papillary thyroid carcinoma) tyrosine kinase: roles in specific gene regulation and cellular transformation. Mol Endocrinol. 2003;17:1155–66.
43. Kim YR, Byun HS, Won M, et al. Modulatory role of phospholipase D in the activation of signal transducer and activator of transcription (STAT)-3 by thyroid oncogenic kinase RET/PTC. BMC Cancer. 2008;8:144.
44. Ng YP, Cheung ZH, Ip NY. STAT3 as a downstream mediator of Trk signaling and functions. J Biol Chem. 2006;281:15636–44.
45. Powell Jr DJ, Russell J, Nibu K, et al. The RET/PTC3 oncogene: metastatic solid-type papillary carcinomas in murine thyroids. Cancer Res. 1998;58:5523–8.
46. Nikiforova MN, Kimura ET, Gandhi M, et al. BRAF mutations in thyroid tumors are restricted to papillary carcinomas and anaplastic or poorly differentiated carcinomas arising from papillary carcinomas. J Clin Endocrinol Metab. 2003;88:5399–404.
47. Nikiforova MN, Nikiforov YE. Molecular genetics of thyroid cancer: implications for diagnosis, treatment and prognosis. Expert Rev Mol Diagn. 2008;8:83–95.
48. Knauf JA, Ma X, Smith EP, et al. Targeted expression of BRAF[V600E] in thyroid cells of transgenic mice results in papillary thyroid cancers that undergo dedifferentiation. Cancer Res. 2005;65:4238–45.
49. Faustino A, Couto JP, Pópulo H, et al. mTOR pathway overactivation in BRAF mutated papillary thyroid carcinoma. Clin Endocrinol Metab. 2012;97:E1139–49.

50. Xing M. Genetic alterations in the phosphatidylinositol-3 kinase/Akt pathway in thyroid cancer. Thyroid. 2010;20:697–706.
51. Nikiforov YE. Molecular diagnostics of thyroid tumors. Arch Pathol Lab Med. 2011;135:569–77.
52. Vasko V, Espinosa AV, Scouten W, et al. Gene expression and functional evidence of epithelial-to-mesenchymal transition in papillary thyroid carcinoma invasion. Proc Natl Acad Sci USA. 2007;104:2803–8.
53. Knauf JA, Sartor MA, Medvedovic M, et al. Progression of BRAF-induced thyroid cancer is associated with epithelial-mesenchymal transition requiring concomitant MAP kinase and TGFβ signaling. Oncogene. 2011;30:3153–62.
54. Tiwari N, Gheldof A, Tatari M, et al. EMT as the ultimate survival mechanism of cancer cells. Semin Cancer Biol. 2012;22:194–207.
55. Mazeh H. MicroRNA as a diagnostic tool in fine-needle aspiration biopsy of thyroid nodules. Oncologist. 2012;17:1032–8.
56. Brait M, Loyo M, Rosenbaum E, et al. Correlation between BRAF mutation and promoter methylation of TIMP3, RARP2 and RASSF1A in thyroid cancer. Epigenetics. 2012;7:710–9.
57. Marotta V, Guerra A, Sapio MR, et al. RET/PTC rearrangement in benign and malignant thyroid diseases: a clinical standpoint. Eur J Endocrinol. 2011;165:499–507.
58. Romei C, Elisei R. RET/PTC translocations and clinico-pathological features in human papillary thyroid carcinoma. Front Endocrinol (Lausanne). 2012;3:54.
59. Kim TH, Park YJ, Lim JA, et al. The association of the BRAF (V600E) mutation with prognostic factors and poor clinical outcome in papillary thyroid cancer: a meta-analysis. Cancer. 2012;118:1764–73.
60. Tufano RP, Teixeira GV, Bishop J, et al. RAF mutation in papillary thyroid cancer and its value in tailoring initial treatment: a systematic review and meta-analysis. Medicine (Baltimore). 2012;91:274–86.
61. Basolo F, Torregrossa L, Giannini R, et al. Correlation between the BRAF V600E mutation and tumor invasiveness in papillary thyroid carcinomas smaller than 20 millimeters: analysis of 1060 cases. J Clin Endocrinol Metab. 2010;95:4197–205.
62. Rodrigues HG, de Pontes AA, Adan LF. Use of molecular markers in samples obtained from preoperative aspiration of thyroid. Endocr J. 2012;59:417–24.
63. Adeniran AJ, Zhu Z, Gandhi M, et al. Correlation between genetic alterations and microscopic features, clinical manifestations, and prognostic characteristics of thyroid papillary carcinomas. Am J Surg Pathol. 2006;30:216–22.
64. Motoi N, Sakamoto A, Yamochi T, et al. Role of ras mutation in the progression of thyroid carcinoma of follicular epithelial origin. Pathol Res Pract. 2000;196:1–7.
65. Esapa CT, Johnson SJ, Kendall-Taylor P, et al. Prevalence of Ras mutations in thyroid neoplasia. Clin Endocrinol (Oxf). 1999;50:529–35.
66. Basolo F, Pisaturo F, Pollina LE, et al. N-ras mutation in poorly differentiated thyroid carcinomas: correlation with bone metastases and inverse correlation to thyroglobulin expression. Thyroid. 2000;10:19–23.
67. Myers MB, McKim KL, Parsons BL. A subset of papillary thyroid carcinomas contain KRAS mutant subpopulations at levels above normal thyroid. Mol Carcinog. 2014;53:159–67.
68. Sahin M, Allard BL, Yates M, et al. PPARgamma staining as a surrogate for PAX8/PPARgamma fusion oncogene expression in follicular neoplasms: clinicopathological correlation and histopathological diagnostic value. J Clin Endocrinol Metab. 2005;90:463–8.
69. Mehta V, Nikiforov YE, Ferris RL. Use of molecular biomarkers in FNA specimens to personalize treatment for thyroid surgery. Head Neck. 2013;35:1499–506.
70. Ferraz C, Eszlinger M, Paschke R. Current state and future perspective of molecular diagnosis of fine-needle aspiration biopsy of thyroid nodules. J Clin Endocrinol Metab. 2011;96:2016–26.
71. Nikiforov YE, Ohori NP, Hodak SP, et al. Impact of mutational testing on the diagnosis and management of patients with cytologically indeterminate thyroid nodules: a prospective analysis of 1056 FNA samples. J Clin Endocrinol Metab. 2011;96:3390–7.
72. Filicori F, Keutgen XM, Buitrago D, et al. Risk stratification of indeterminate thyroid fine-needle aspiration biopsy specimens based on mutation analysis. Surgery. 2011;150:1085–91.

73. Marques AR, Espadinha C, Catarino AL, et al. Expression of PAX8-PPARγ1 rearrangements in both follicular thyroid carcinomas and adenomas. J Clin Endocrinol Metab. 2002;87:3947–52.
74. Moses W, Weng J, Sansano I, et al. Molecular testing for somatic mutations improves the accuracy of thyroid fine-needle aspiration biopsy. World J Surg. 2010;34:2589–94.
75. Cantara S, Capezzone M, Marchisotta S, et al. Impact of proto-oncogene mutation detection in cytological specimens from thyroid nodules improves the diagnostic accuracy of cytology. J Clin Endocrinol Metab. 2010;95:1365–9.
76. Griffith OL, Melck A, Jones SJM, et al. Meta-analysis and meta-review of thyroid cancer gene expression profiling studies identifies important diagnostic biomarkers. J Clin Oncol. 2006;24:5043–51.
77. Kebebew E, Peng M, Reiff E, et al. ECM1 and TMPRSS4 are diagnostic markers of malignant thyroid neoplasms and improve the accuracy of fine needle aspiration biopsy. Ann Surg. 2005;242:353–61; discussion 361–3.
78. Kebebew E, Peng M, Reiff E, et al. Diagnostic and prognostic value of cell-cycle regulatory genes in malignant thyroid neoplasms. World J Surg. 2006;30:767–74.
79. Rosen J, He M, Umbricht C, et al. A six-gene model for differentiating benign from malignant thyroid tumors on the basis of gene expression. Surgery. 2005;138:1050–6; discussion 1056–7.
80. Cerutti JM. Employing genetic markers to improve diagnosis of thyroid tumor fine needle biopsy. Curr Genomics. 2011;12:589–96.
81. Prasad NB, Kowalski J, Tsai HL, et al. Three-gene molecular diagnostic model for thyroid cancer. Thyroid. 2012;22:275–84.
82. Hodak SP, Rosenthal DS, American Thyroid Association Clinical Affairs Committee. Information for clinicians: commercially available molecular diagnosis testing in the evaluation of thyroid nodule FNA specimens. Thyroid. 2013;23:131–4.
83. Walsh PS, Wilde JI, Tom EY, et al. Analytical performance verification of a molecular diagnostic for cytology-indeterminate thyroid nodules. J Clin Endocrinol Metab. 2012;97:E2297–306.
84. Alexander EK, Kennedy GC, Baloch ZW, et al. Preoperative diagnosis of benign thyroid nodules with indeterminate cytology. N Engl J Med. 2012;367:705–15.
85. Chiu CG, Strugnell SS, Griffith OL. Diagnostic utility of galectin-3 in thyroid cancer. Am J Pathol. 2010;176:206–7.
86. Kouniavsky G, Zeiger MA. The quest for diagnostic molecular markers for thyroid nodules with indeterminate or suspicious cytology. J Surg Oncol. 2012;105:438–43.
87. de Matos LL, Del Giglio AB, Matsubayashi CO, et al. Expression of ck-19, galectin-3 and hbme-1 in the differentiation of thyroid lesions: systematic review and diagnostic meta-analysis. Diagn Pathol. 2012;7:97.
88. Carpi A, Naccarato AG, Iervasi G, et al. Large needle aspiration biopsy and galectin-3 determination in selected thyroid nodules with indeterminate FNA-cytology. Br J Cancer. 2006;95:204–9.
89. Leonardi GC, Candido S, Carbone M, et al. MicroRNAs and thyroid cancer: biological and clinical significance (Review). Int J Mol Med. 2012;30:991–9.
90. Kitano M, Rahbari R, Patterson EE, et al. Evaluation of candidate diagnostic microRNAs in thyroid fine-needle aspiration biopsy samples. Thyroid. 2012;22:285–91.
91. Vriens MR, Weng J, Suh I, et al. MicroRNA expression profiling is a potential diagnostic tool for thyroid cancer. Cancer. 2012;118:3426–32.
92. de la Chapelle A, Jazdzewski K. MicroRNAs in thyroid cancer. J Clin Endocrinol Metab. 2011;96:3326–36.
93. Keutgen XM, Filicori F, Crowley MJ, et al. A panel of four miRNAs accurately differentiates malignant from benign indeterminate thyroid lesions on fine needle aspiration. Clin Cancer Res. 2012;18:2032–8.
94. Mazeh H, Levy Y, Mizrahi I, et al. Differentiating benign from malignant thyroid nodules using micro ribonucleic acid amplification in residual cells obtained by fine needle aspiration biopsy. J Surg Res. 2013;180:216–21.
95. Shen R, Liyanarachchi S, Li W, et al. MicroRNA signature in thyroid fine needle aspiration cytology applied to 'atypia of undetermined significance' cases. Thyroid. 2012;22:9–16.

The Significance of Cervical Lymph Nodes in Well-Differentiated Thyroid Cancer

2

Richard W. Nason and K. Alok Pathak

Introduction

Well-differentiated thyroid cancer (WDTC), papillary thyroid cancer (PTC) and follicular thyroid cancer (FTC) are relatively rare. In 2012, a total of 5,600 new cases of thyroid cancer were diagnosed in Canada. Death from thyroid cancer is an even rarer event, with <400 recorded deaths in the same year [1]. To put this in perspective, breast cancer accounted for 22,900 new cases and 5,200 deaths. WDTC has a good prognosis with minimal morbidity if treated properly. Adequate initial surgery offers the most useful contribution to both overall and relapse survival for WDTC. The extent of this surgery has generated controversy for decades and this controversy includes the indications and extent of surgery for cervical lymph nodes. The challenge in the management of this malignancy is to tailor the treatment to be aggressive enough to eradicate the disease, but not so excessive as to cause unnecessary morbidity.

R.W. Nason (✉)
Head and Neck Surgical Oncology, CancerCare Manitoba,
675 McDermott Ave, Winnipeg, MB R3E0V9, Canada
e-mail: nasonrw@cc.umanitoba.ca

K.A. Pathak
Head and Neck Surgical Oncology, CancerCare Manitoba, University of Manitoba,
675 McDermott Ave, Winnipeg, MB R3E0V9, Canada
e-mail: alok.pathak@cancercare.mb.ca

© K. Alok Pathak, Richard W. Nason, Janice L. Pasieka, Rehan Kazi,
Raghav C. Dwivedi 2015
Springer India/Byword Books
K.A. Pathak et al. (eds.), *Management of Thyroid Cancer: Special Considerations*,
Head and Neck Cancer Clinics, DOI 10.1007/978-81-322-2434-1_2

Natural History of WDTC

Along with being relatively rare, thyroid cancer has an indolent course or a long natural history. In a frequently cited retrospective review by Mazzaferri and Jhiang of 1,355 patients with a median follow up of 15.7 years, 289 recurrences and 70 disease-related deaths were reported [2]. Slightly more than one-half of the recurrences and just shy of one-half of the deaths occurred by 5 years. Tumour recurrences and cancer deaths continued to occur sporadically over the 40-year time span of this study. Similar data are reported by Cady et al., in which approximately one-half of all recurrences and deaths occurred after 5 years [3]. In this series, tumour recurrences and death occurred sporadically in ≤25 and 30 years, respectively. In a series from Institute Gustave Roussy, 25 % of first recurrences were diagnosed after 25 years [4].

The recurrence rate for WDTC approximates 20 % and is most frequently identified in the neck, followed by the thyroid bed and distant metastases [2, 5, 6]. The most frequent site of distant metastases is the lung, followed by bone [2, 5]. For FTC, distant metastases are the more frequent site of initial recurrence [2, 3].

The mortality rate for WDTC in North America is ~11 %; it approaches 20 % in Europe [6]. Disease-specific mortality is distributed between local recurrence with airway obstruction and distant metastases, with a bias to the former in most series [2, 5, 7–9]

As a result of this low incidence, protracted course, low mortality rates, and the influence of other variables, notably age on outcome, prospective randomized trials to resolve controversies in the management of this disease are felt by many to be impractical. Statistical end-points, such as recurrence or survival, are relatively infrequent and distributed over a long time span. In brief, WDTC kills relatively infrequently. The nature of this disease allows for great variability in treatment methods without any appreciable change in mortality. The effect of any one treatment therefore becomes difficult to assess [10].

Incidence and Patterns of Cervical Lymph Node Involvement

Although the majority of thyroid cancer cases present with a thyroid nodule, 15–30 % of patients present with a palpably enlarged lymph node [11–13]. Regional node metastases, at least microscopic involvement, occur most commonly with PTC and ranges from 30 to 90 % of cases, with a 30–40 % incidence of clinically evident lymph node metastases at presentation [6, 11, 12, 14]. The higher incidence is recorded in series in which lymph node dissections have been done on an elective or prophylactic basis [2, 7, 15, 16]. FTC, classically associated with distant metastases by haematogenous spread, generally exhibits a lower incidence of cervical metastases—in the range of 10–15 % [17]. The incidence of metastases in PTC appears to be related to the age of the patient. Nodal metastases are far more common in patients of <40 years age, and are strikingly predominant in the paediatric population, being present in 60–90 % of cases [18]. Men harbour lymph node metastases more frequently than women [19]. A relationship between tumour size and cumulative risk of metastases has been identified and multifocal cancers are more likely to have nodal metastases [20–25]. Molecular markers to predict clinically significant lymph node metastases might play a role in the future [19, 25].

Frazell and Foote were one of the first to report the frequency and distribution of involved lymph nodes in 182 radical neck dissection specimens [7]. When a neck dissection was done electively, involvement of lymph nodes was identified in 61.2 % of cases. Patients with no clinical evidence of cervical metastases were 4 times more likely to have their metastases limited to a single area than those showing some clinical signs of local metastases. When the frequency of involvement of various node baring areas was examined, involvement of the lateral neck and spinal accessory chain appeared to be more frequent when lymph nodes were palpable. Six per cent of patients with clinically negative necks had involvement of the spinal accessory nodes versus 36 % with clinically palpable adenopathy. Noguchi et al., based on the observation that the para tracheal area was most frequently involved in the majority of patients with a single metastatic deposit, suggested that the pattern of nodal metastases in the early stages of thyroid cancer was directed downwards and laterally in the central compartment [16]. He emphasized, as had Frazell and Foote [7], that the rate of lymph node metastases was not only high in the paratracheal region but also in the lateral neck. Quabain et al. designed a study to identify the precise localization of lymph node micrometastases and map their cervical involvement in relation to tumour location within the thyroid gland [26]. When thyroid carcinoma was located in the upper third of the thyroid lobe, the lymph node metastases were found in the direction of upward lymphatic flow. When the tumour was located in the lower third or isthmus lymph node, micrometastases were directed downwards. In addition, micrometastases did not cross the midline but remained in the ipsilateral side of the tumour.

Gimm et al. divided the lymph node metastases into cervicocentral and cervicolateral groups [27]. In a review of 35 patients with bilateral thyroidectomy and neck dissection, the authors noted that the ipsilateral cervicocentral compartment was involved in 24 and the ipsilateral cervicolateral compartment in 19 patients. Contralateral cervicocentral metastases were observed in 5 patients with larger primary Amours. No involvement was evident of the contralateral cervicolateral compartment. Machens and coworkers described similar findings in 134 neck dissections [20]. They described the incidence of lymph node metastases at the time of primary surgery and at the time of re-operation. The incidence of metastases was as follows:

(i) in the ipsilateral cervicocentral compartment 29 % and 34 %, respectively;
(ii) in the contralateral cervicocentral compartment 13 % and 15 %, respectively;
(iii) in the ipsilateral cervicolateral compartment 29 % and 21 %, respectively;
(iv) in the contralateral cervicolateral compartment 3 % and 18 %, respectively; and
(v) in the mediastinal 0 % and 3 %, respectively. Contralateral cervicolateral and mediastinal compartments are rarely affected by PTC. Gimm et al. also

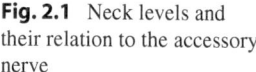

Fig. 2.1 Neck levels and
their relation to the accessory
nerve

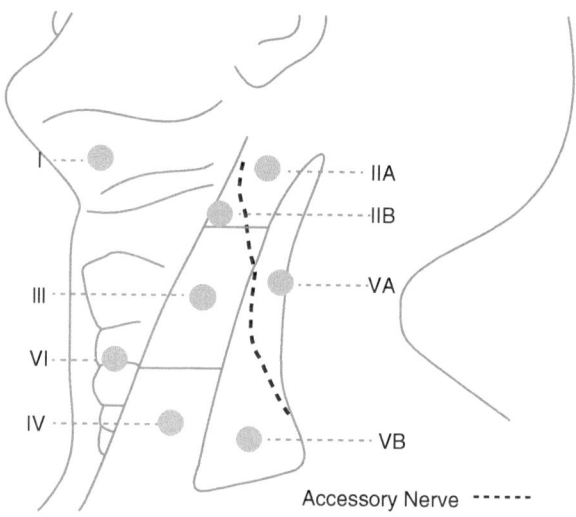

noted that the caudal portions of the cervical lateral compartment were
involved more frequently than the cranial compartment [27]. They emphasized that the initial lymphatic flow was from the thyroid gland to the ipsilateral lower jugular lymph nodes and venous angle. Others have
emphasized the frequent involvement of both the central and lateral compartments [23, 28–32].

Sivanandan and Soo [33] were the first to describe metastases from papillary
carcinoma of the thyroid by neck level [19, 34] (Fig. 2.1). They described the distribution of lymph node metastases in 75 patients undergoing 85 therapeutic neck
dissections [33]. This study did not address the central compartment. Fourteen specimens showed only a single level of involvement. Levels II, III and IV were at the
greatest risk of metastatic disease. Level III was the most consistently involved,
followed by level IV and then level II. Level V was not likely to be involved and
level I nodes were seen only with extensive neck disease. Levels I and V nodes were
never seen in isolation, i.e. they only occurred with involvement of other levels.
Other descriptions of lymph node involvement in the lateral neck after a therapeutic
neck dissection by level are summarized in Table 2.1.
Sivanandan and Soo noted involvement of multiple levels in 84 % of their specimens [33]. In other series multiple levels were involved in 60–80 % of patients [35,
36]. Eighty-one per cent of patients presenting after an excisional biopsy were noted
to have additional nodes [36]. Discontinual nodal metastases (skip metastases),
defined as lateral lymph node metastases in the absence of central lymph node
metastases, occurs in 7–19 % of patients [16, 25, 36–38]. With unilateral primary
tumours the incidence of contralateral disease in the central and lateral compartments is low, in the order of 0–15 % [20–22, 27, 39, 40]. Ahmadi and co-workers
examined the distribution of nodal metastases in primary and recurrent disease;
level IV was more commonly involved in recurrent cases [41].

Table 2.1 Incidence and distribution of lymph node metastases by level in patients undergoing a therapeutic lateral neck dissection for papillary thyroid cancer

References	n	Neck level (% involvement)					Comments
		I	II	III	IV	V	
Pingpank et al. (2002) [36]	51	12	43	76	59	26	Level I dissected in 31 %
Kupferman et al. (2004) [35]	39	14	52	53	41	21	Level I dissected in 7 %
Kupferman et al. (2008) [24]	70	27	57	62	62	53	Level I neck dissection in 43 %
Yanir and Doweck (2008) [22]	27	–	54	68	57	20	level I not dissected
Farrag et al. (2009) [42]	53	–	60	66	50	40	Level I not dissected
Yuce et al. (2009) [38]	46	–	46	69	66	34	Level I not dissected
Spriano et al. (2009) [39]	77	1	38	45	52	8	Level I neck dissection in 38 %; level V dissected in 69 %
Lim et al. (2010) [76]	70	–	49	74	69	16	Level I not dissected
Nam et al. (2012) [77]	50	0	40	46	42	10	Level I dissected

Recent studies have focused on the involvement of lymph nodes adjacent to the accessory nerve in the anterior triangle (level II) and posterior triangle (level V) [36, 40, 42, 43]. Level II is subdivided by the accessory nerve with the portion above and behind the nerve designated as level IIb (Fig. 2.1) [19]. Pingpank and co-workers noted metastases to level IIb in 7 (21 %) of 34 neck dissections [36]. In 3 patients level IIb was the only site of level II involvement. Farrag et al. [42] and Lee et al. [43] described positive nodes in this area in 11.8 and 7 % of dissections, and in both series level IIa was always involved. Level V is subdivided by a plane defined by the inferior border of the cricoid cartilage into level Va superiorly and level Vb inferiorly [19]. Level Va contains the nodes surrounding the accessory nerve. In studies, in which level V has been subdivided, no nodes have been identified in level Va [40, 42].

In summary, based on the surgical management of thyroid cancer, and the surgical and pathological anatomy, two generally accepted anatomical compartments exist—a central compartment and the median visceral compartment, which lies between the trachea and carotid arteries from the hyoid bone to the brachial cephalic vein (level VI). This compartment contains the preglandular nodes, pretracheal nodes, paratracheal nodes, recurrent chain, and the anterior mediastinal nodes. The superior mediastinal nodes are assigned to level VII. The lateral compartment lies between the carotid artery and trapezius muscle and contains the upper middle and lower jugular nodes and the spinal accessory chain of lymph nodes (levels II-V). Regional lymph node metastases from WDTC are frequent and predictable in distribution. The first echelon nodes are the ipsilateral central compartment with subsequent drainage to the lateral neck where metastatic disease is most commonly identified in levels IIb, III, IV and Va. The lymph node metastases are often multiple, and skip metastases are infrequent.

Detection of Cervical Node Metastases and the Role of Diagnostic Imaging

A role for diagnostic imaging in the evaluation of thyroid malignancy has evolved. Examination of the neck is relatively unreliable with reported false-positive and false-negative rates for detection of metastatic disease and nodes of 20–30 % [44, 45]. Imaging studies, including high-resolution ultrasound, CT and MRI are more accurate than physical examination in determining macroscopic node involvement. Current guidelines for the management of WDTC recommend, as the standard, preoperative high-resolution ultrasound of the neck for all patients undergoing thyroid surgery for malignant cytology [19, 46]. The features on ultrasound that are used to determine positive node involvement include size criteria (>13 mm, short access diameter), shape (assessment of the long to short access), and internal architecture (homogeneous and hyperechochic; peripheral punctate calcification; cystic change) [25, 44, 47]. The sensitivity of ultrasound in detecting involved lymph nodes approximates 30 % [48, 49]. Ultrasound is less sensitive to the presence of involved nodes in the central compartment because of the presence of the thyroid gland and the air-filled trachea. [19, 44, 47] Evidence shows that the combined use of ultrasound and CT scan is more accurate than ultrasound alone [47, 50]. Fine-needle aspiration biopsy (FNAB) is appropriate in the evaluation of suspect lymph nodes before surgical management [19]. The iodine load from CT imaging of the neck may alter radioactive iodine uptake in 6 weeks after its administration [44].

Sentinel lymph node biopsy (SLNB) has been evaluated in WDTC [37]. A role for SLNB in WDTC has not been established. In the authors' opinion the value of this technique would be to identify the subset of patients without occult metastases in which case there would be no controversy with respect to elective management of the neck.

In summary, imaging studies are most useful to assess the lateral compartment. The best way to assess the central compartment of the neck remains surgical exploration.

Impact of Cervical Node Metastases on Prognosis

The high frequency of involvement of cervical lymph nodes in WDTC is well established and regional nodes represent the most frequent site of recurrence [2, 12, 31, 51]. An association of cervical lymph nodes with distant metastases has been observed [9, 12, 21, 52]. It would seem that it should be relatively easy to demonstrate an adverse influence of regional node disease on survival. This has not been the case. The relative, independent and reproducible risk factors for survival, as defined by the EORTC [53] and subsequently the AGES [54], AMES [55] and MACIS [56] prognostic scoring systems, and confirmed in other large retrospective reviews [57, 58], are few. The most consistently important variables influencing survival from differentiated thyroid cancer are advanced age (>45 or 50 years), and the presence of distant metastases. Size and extra-thyroidal extension seem to be reproducible independent variables but with less influence on survival than the first two variables. These variables would not appear to be controversial. Note that regional metastases are not included.

The overall impact of cervical metastases on survival is probably small. Initial reports showed conflicting evidence. It has been observed that the presence of nodal metastases had no effect on either recurrence or survival [3, 55, 58, 59]. Others suggested that lymph node metastases, as they are associated with a higher rate of recurrence, exercise a significant influence on survival [2, 12, 21, 60, 61]. The impact on survival in these series could be attributed to the longer period of follow-up; however, these studies did not adjust the survival analysis by age.

Hughes et al. presented the results of a matched pair analysis comparing 100 patients with lymph node metastases to 100 patients without [62]. They compared ipsilateral N1 nodal disease with those without nodal disease to examine the significance of nodal spread in patients with otherwise equivalent prognostic factors. The 20-year disease-specific survival rates in the N1 and N0 groups were 92 % and 93 %, respectively. Although it did not reach significance, the 20-year survival rate of N1 patients older than 45 years was lower (70 %) than the 20-year survival rates of the age-matched N0 patients (90 %). The overall recurrence rate did not reach significance—17 % and 11 % in N1 and N0 patients, respectively. Age had a major influence in the incidence of disease recurrence, with an 8 % incidence of recurrence in the younger patients, compared with 31 % in the older patients. The authors concluded that the presence of nodal disease was not a significant prognostic factor in patients overall, but its presence did influence a risk of tumour recurrence and mortality in the older patient [62]. Lundgren et al. reported a nested case–control study of a cohort of 5,123 patients with differentiated thyroid cancer treated in Sweden from 1958 to 1987 [63]. The patients were matched by age, gender and calendar period. The mean follow up was 6.7 years. Patients with lymph node metastases experienced a higher mortality (HR 2.5; 95 % CI 1.6–4.1).

A subset of patients with WDTC and node metastases seem to do worse. Older patients are one group, as initially noted by Cady et al. [3] Shaha et al., using a multivariate model, showed that positive nodes significantly influenced survival in patients older than 45 years [64]. Others noted that the prognosis for survival was worse in older node-positive patients [21, 31, 61, 65]. Decreased survival has been associated with mediastinal nodes [2, 31], bilateral nodes [2], a node size of >3 cm [66–68], and extracapsular extension [67]. Simpson and co-workers, in a Canadian survey of 1,074 PTCs and 504 FTCs, found that nodal involvement influenced prognosis in FTC, but not PTC [69].

Leaving aside overall survival, there seems to be a more consistent agreement that the presence of positive lymph nodes does influence recurrence. Leboulleux et al. identified palpable lymph nodes as a significant risk factor for disease recurrence [70]. Other factors associated with recurrence in this series included the number of lymph nodes (>10), extracellular extension, and positive thyroglobulin at 6 months with T4 withdrawal. Wada et al., using a multivariate model in 134 patients with 42 therapeutic and 92 elective neck dissections, established that lymphadenopathy at the time of presentation was significantly related to recurrence [23]. Again, it was observed that local recurrence was impacted by the number of positive lymph nodes. Beasley et al. in a series of 347 patients with stages I and II disease noted that neck node metastases impacted disease-free survival on multivariate analysis [71]. Patients with lateral lymph nodes, multiple level involvement, and superior mediastinal involvement had a worse outcome than those with central compartment involvement alone. The influence of positive nodes at the time of presentation on recurrence has been emphasized in other series [2, 12, 21, 27, 62, 65]. Randolph and co-workers recently challenged the paradigm of assigning the same magnitude of risk to all patients with N1 disease [72]. In their study, the recurrence rate for patients staged N0 at presentation was 2 % compared with 22 % for those who are initially N-positive. They noted that in pN1 patients the recurrence rate was impacted by the number of positive nodes—4 % with <5 nodes and 19 % with >5 nodes. Extranodal extension was associated with a median risk of recurrence of 24 % [72]. A scoring system to stratify patients by risk of lymph node recurrence has been proposed by Ito and co-workers [73]. One point each was assigned to the following: (i) age of >55 years; (ii) male gender; (iii) massive extrathyroidal extension; and (iv) tumour of >3 cm diameter. The 10-year regional disease-free survival was 98.4 % with a score of 0. Survival decreased incrementally to 64.7 % with a score of 4. The use of molecular markers may help predict recurrence in the future [74].

In summary, the predominant opinion today is that local node metastases increases the risk of local recurrence and cancer-specific mortality in older patients (>45 years), especially if the nodes are bilateral, involvement of mediastinal nodes, and if the nodes are fixed, or if there is tumour invasion through the capsule of the lymph node [46]. This notion is reflected in the staging system for thyroid cancer, in which for patients 45 years or older, the presence of lymph node metastases (N1) upgrades stage I or II to stage III [75]. Despite the frequency of microscopic lymph node involvement (60–90 %) only 5–15 % of patients with PTC in whom no prophylactic neck dissection has been performed develop clinically significant lymph node metastases at a later date [25].

An Overview of Management

Careful and appropriate surgery is the most important component in the treatment of WDTC. The extent of surgical resection depends on the extent of cancer with the aim to control the cancer and avoid re-operation, if possible with minimal morbidity. Badly treated thyroid cancer can be a progressive and recurrent disease, whereas with expert management it is readily controlled. Local recurrence and complications of surgery are equally important in determining the timing and extent of treatment of the neck. For this reason the management of the central and lateral compartments of the neck is considered separately. Current guidelines for the management of the neck in patients with WDTC are shown in Table 2.2.

Table 2.2 Guidelines for the treatment of the neck in WDTC

Central compartment (level VI) Recommendation 27	Lateral compartment (levels II-V) Recommendation 28
(a) Therapeutic central compartment (level VI) neck dissection for patients with clinically involved central or lateral neck lymph nodes should accompany total thyroidectomy to provide clearance of the disease from the central neck. Recommendation rating: B	Therapeutic lateral compartment lymph node dissection should be performed for patients with biopsy-proven metastatic lateral cervical lymphadenopathy. Recommendation rating: B
(b) Prophylactic central compartment neck dissection (ipsilateral or bilateral) may be performed in patients with papillary thyroid carcinoma with clinically uninvolved central neck lymph nodes, especially for advanced primary tumours (T3 or T4). Recommendation rating: C	
(c) Near-total or total thyroidectomy without prophylactic central neck dissection might be appropriate for small (T1 or T2), noninvasive, clinically node-negative PTCs and most follicular cancers. Recommendation rating: C	

Adapted from the American Thyroid Association Management Guidelines for Patients with Thyroid Nodules and Differentiated Thyroid Cancer (Cooper 2009) [46]

Summary

WDTC has an indolent course and a relatively good prognosis in most patients. There are a limited number of 'statistical' end-points, recurrence or death, to assess in this disease. As prospective studies to base treatment decisions are lacking, strict treatment guidelines are inappropriate. Although associated with a good overall prognosis, the disease is fatal in a small proportion of patients. The claim that WDTC is a 'benign disease' is untrue. Most patients with differentiated thyroid cancer, especially of the papillary type, have lymph node metastases to some extent at diagnosis. One of the most consistent features of PTC is its capacity for regional metastases of the lymph nodes. The influence of lymph node metastases in PTC on survival is minor. This may be of more significance in the highrisk or older patient. The presence of lymph node metastasis does influence recurrence. Nodes beget nodes. Careful surgery is the most important component in the treatment of this disease. The extent of surgical resection should depend on the extent of cancer, with the aim to control the cancer and avoid re-operation, if possible with minimal morbidity. Badly treated thyroid cancer can be a progressive and recurrent disease whereas with expert management it is readily controlled. Local or regional recurrence and complications of surgery are equally important in determining the definitive extent of the procedure. The management of the neck is best considered in relation to the cervical central and cervical lateral compartments. Elective or prophylactic neck dissection of the central compartment is now recommended and supported by many investigators. The major argument presented for this is a high incidence of metastatic disease to the central compartment, a relatively low risk of complications with elective dissection, and a relatively high risk of complications with re-operation of the central compartment. Opponents of routine prophylactic dissection of the central compartment argue that there is no evidence of a survival benefit. They also argue that re-operation can be done relatively safely. Prophylactic or elective neck dissection of the lateral compartment is not supported at present. It is generally felt that morbidity does not increase with treatment of metachronous disease in this compartment. In both prophylactic and therapeutic neck dissections, the classic radical neck dissection has been replaced by compartment-oriented and level-specific neck dissections, which emphasize preservation of function. Limited node picking, 'berry picking' procedures are generally not accepted as they lead to an unacceptable rate of recurrence. The more comprehensive neck dissections may preclude a need for additional operations for recurrence associated with an increased risk of complications. The lateral cervical nodes appear to be less critical to recurrence and survival than nodal involvement in the central compartment.

References

1. Canadian Cancer Society. Canada cancer statistics 2012. http://www.cancer.ca/Canada.
2. Mazzaferri EL, Jhiang SM. Long-term impact of initial surgical and medical therapy on papillary and follicular thyroid cancer. Am J Med. 1994;97:418–28.
3. Cady B, Sedgwick CE, Meissner A, et al. Risk factor analysis in differentiated thyroid cancer. Cancer. 1979;43:810–20.
4. Tubiana M, Schlumberger M, Rougier P, et al. Long-term results and prognostic factors in patients with differentiated thyroid carcinoma. Cancer. 1985;55:794–804.
5. Samaan NA, Schultz PN, Hickey RC, et al. The results of various modalities of treatment of well-differentiated thyroid carcinoma: a retrospective review of 1599 patients. J Clin Endocrinol Metab. 1992;75:714–20.
6. McConahey WM, Hay ID, Woolner LB, et al. Papillary thyroid cancer treated at the Mayo Clinic, 1946 through 1970: initial manifestations, pathologic findings, therapy and outcome. Mayo Clin Proc. 1986;61:978–96.
7. Frazell EL, Foote Jr FW. Papillary thyroid carcinoma: pathological findings in cases with and without clinical evidence of cervical node involvement. Cancer. 1955;8:1164–6.
8. Tennvall J, Björklund A, Moller T, et al. Is the EORTC prognostic index of thyroid cancer valid in differentiated thyroid carcinoma? Retrospective multivariate analysis of differentiated thyroid carcinoma with long follow-up. Cancer. 1986;57:1405–14.
9. Carcangiu ML, Zampi G, Pupi A, et al. Papillary carcinoma of the thyroid. A clinicopathologic study of 241 cases treated at the University of Florence, Italy. Cancer. 1985;55:805–28.
10. Hutter RV, Frazell EL, Foote Jr FW. Elective radical neck dissection: an assessment of its use in the management of papillary thyroid cancer. CA Cancer J Clin. 1970;20:87–93.
11. Mazzaferri EL, Young RL. Papillary thyroid carcinoma: a 10 year follow-up report of the impact of therapy in 576 patients. Am J Med. 1981;70:511–8.
12. McHenry CR, Rosen IB, Walfish PG. Prospective management of nodal metastases in differentiated thyroid cancer. Am J Surg. 1991;162:353–6.
13. Sanders LE, Rossi RL. Occult well differentiated thyroid carcinoma presenting as cervical node disease. World J Surg. 1995;19:642–7.
14. Cady B, Sedgwick CE, Meissner WA, et al. Changing clinical, pathologic, therapeutic, and survival patterns in differentiated thyroid carcinoma. Ann Surg. 1976;184:541–53.

15. Attie JN, Khafif RA, Steckler RM. Elective neck dissection in papillary carcinoma of the thyroid. Am J Surg. 1971;122:464–71.
16. Noguchi S, Noguchi A, Murakami N. Papillary carcinoma of the thyroid I. Developing pattern of metastasis. Cancer. 1970;26:1053–60.
17. Harness J, Thompson N, McCleod M, et al. Follicular carcinoma of the thyroid. Trends and treatment. Surgery. 1984;96:972–80.
18. Frankenthaler RA, Sellin RV, Cangir A, et al. Lymph node metastasis from papillary-follicular thyroid carcinoma in young patients. Am J Surg. 1990;160:341–3.
19. Stack B, Ferris R, Goldenberg D. American thyroid association consensus review and statement regarding the anatomy, terminology, and rationale for lateral neck dissection in differentiated thyroid cancer. Thyroid. 2012;22:501–8.
20. Machens A, Hinze R, Thomusch O, et al. Pattern of nodal metastasis for primary and reoperative thyroid cancer. World J Surg. 2002;26:22–8.
21. Scheumann GFW, Gimm O, Wegener G, et al. Prognostic significance and surgical management of locoregional lymph node metastases in papillary thyroid cancer. World J Surg. 1994;18:559–67; discussion 567–8.
22. Yanir Y, Doweck I. Regional metastases in well-differentiated thyroid carcinoma: pattern of spread. Laryngoscope. 2008;118:433–6.
23. Wada N, Duh QY, Sugino K, et al. Lymph node metastasis from 259 papillary thyroid microcarcinomas. Frequency, pattern of occurrence and recurrence, and optimal strategy for neck dissection. Ann Surg. 2003;237:399–407.
24. Kupferman M, Weinstock Y, Santillan A. Predictors of level V metastases in well differentiated thyroid cancer. Head Neck. 2008;30:1469–74.
25. Dionigi G, Dionigi R, Bartalena L, et al. Surgery of lymph nodes in papillary thyroid cancer. Expert Rev Anticancer Ther. 2006;6:1217–9.
26. Quabain S, Nakano S, Baba M, et al. Distribution of lymph node metastases in pN0 well-differentiated thyroid carcinoma. Surgery. 2002;131:249–56.
27. Gimm O, Rath FW, Dralle H. Pattern of lymph node metastases in papillary thyroid carcinoma. Br J Surg. 1998;85:252–4.
28. Ardito G, Revelli L, Tosti F, et al. Surgery of differentiated thyroid carcinoma, lymph node metastases and locoregional recurrence. Rays. 2000;25:199–206.
29. Noguchi S, Murakami N. The value of lymph-node dissection in patients with differentiated thyroid cancer. Surg Clin North Am. 1987;67:251–61.
30. Ozaki O, Ito K, Kobayashi K, et al. Modified neck dissection for patients with nonadvanced, differentiated carcinoma of the thyroid. World J Surg. 1988;12:825–9.
31. Coburn M, Wanebo HJ. Prognostic factors and management considerations in patients with cervical metastases of thyroid cancer. Am J Surg. 1992;164:671–6.
32. Marcheta FC, Sako K, Matsuura H. Modified neck dissection for carcinoma of the thyroid gland. Am J Surg. 1970;120:452–5.
33. Sivanandan R, Soo KC. Pattern of cervical lymph node metastases from papillary carcinoma of the thyroid. Br J Surg. 2001;88:1241–4.
34. Ferlito A, Robbins KT, Shah JP, et al. Proposal for a rational classification of neck dissections. Head Neck. 2011;33:445–50.
35. Kupferman ME, Patterson M, Mandel SJ, et al. Patterns of lateral neck metastasis in papillary thyroid carcinoma. Arch Otolaryngol Head Neck Surg. 2004;130:857–60.
36. Pingpank Jr JF, Sasson AR, Hanlon AL, et al. Tumor above the spinal accessory nerve in papillary thyroid cancer that involves lateral neck nodes. Arch Otolaryngol Head Neck Surg. 2002;128:1275–8.
37. Pasieka JL. Sentinel lymph node biopsy in the management of thyroid disease. Br J Surg. 2001;88:321–2.
38. Yüce I, Cağh S, Bayram A. Regional metastatic pattern of papillary thyroid carcinoma. Eur Arch Otorhinolaryngol. 2010;267:437–41.
39. Spriano G, Ruscito P, Pellini R, et al. Pattern of regional metastases and prognostic factors in differentiated thyroid carcinoma. Acta Otorhinolaryngol Ital. 2009;29:312–6.

40. Roh J, Kim J, Park C. Central cervical nodal metastases from papillary thyroid microcarcinoma: pattern and factors predictive of nodal metastasis. Ann Surg Oncol. 2008;15:2482–6.
41. Ahmadi N, Grewal A, Davidson BJ. Patterns of cervical lymph node metastases in primary and recurrent papillary thyroid cancer. J Oncol. 2011;2011:735678.
42. Farrag T, Fin F, Brownlee N, et al. Is routine dissection of level II-b and V-a necessary in patients with papillary thyroid cancer undergoing lateral neck dissection for FNA-confirmed metastases in other levels. World J Surg. 2009;33:1680–3.
43. Fee BJ, Wang SG, Lee JC, et al. Level IIb lymph node metastasis in neck dissection for papillary thyroid carcinoma. Arch Otolaryngol Head Neck Surg. 2007;133:1028–30.
44. Watkinson JC, Franklyn JA, Olliff JF. Detection and surgical treatment of cervical lymph nodes in differentiated thyroid cancer. Thyroid. 2006;16:187–94.
45. Ali S, Tiwari R, Snow GB. False-positive and false-negative neck nodes. Head Neck Surg. 1985;8:78–82.
46. American Thyroid Association (ATA) Guidelines Taskforce on Thyroid Nodules and Differentiated Thyroid Cancer, Cooper DS, Doherty GM, Haugen BR, et al. Revised American Thyroid Association management guidelines for patients with thyroid nodules and differentiated thyroid cancer. Thyroid. 2009;19:1167–214.
47. Ito Y, Amino N, Miyauchi A. Thyroid ultrasongraphy. World J Surg. 2010;34:1171–80.
48. Liao S, Shindo M. Management of well differentiated thyroid cancer. Otolaryngol Clin North Am. 2012;45:1163–79.
49. Muller M, Knoefrel W, Gilbertt J, et al. Fateral cervical node metastases in papillary thyrois cancer: a systematic review of imaging-guided and prophylactic removal of the lateral compartment. Clin Endocrinol. 2012;77:126–31.
50. Choi J, Kim J, Kwak J, et al. Preoperative staging of papillary thyroid carcinoma: comparison of ultrasound imaging and CT. AJR Am J Roentgenol. 2009;193:871–8.
51. Wanebo HJ, Andrews W, Kaiser DF. Thyroid cancer: some basic considerations. Am J Surg. 1981;142:474–9.
52. Hay ID, Bergstralh EJ, Grant CS, et al. Impact of primary surgery on outcome in 300 patients with pathologic tumor-node-metastasis stage III papillary thyroid carcinoma treated at one institution from 1940 through 1989. Surgery. 1999;126:1173–81; discussion 1181–2.
53. Byar DP, Green SB, Dor P, et al. A prognostic index for thyroid carcinoma. A study of the E.O.R.T.C. Thyroid Cancer Cooperative Group. Eur J Cancer. 1979;15:1033–41.
54. Hay ID, Grant CS, Taylor WF, et al. Ipsilateral lobectomy versus bilateral lobar resection in papillary thyroid carcinoma: a retrospective analysis of surgical outcome using a novel prognostic scoring system. Surgery. 1987;102:1088–95.
55. Cady B, Rossi R. An expanded view of risk-group definition in differentiated thyroid carcinoma. Surgery. 1988;104:947–53.
56. Hay I, Bergstralh E, Goellner J, et al. Predicting outcome in papillary thyroid carcinoma: development of a reliable prognostic scoring system in a cohort of 1779 patients surgically treated at one institution during 1940 through 1989. Surgery. 1993;114:105–7; discussion 1057–8.
57. DeGroot LJ, Kaplan EL, McCormick M, et al. Natural history, treatment, and course of papillary thyroid carcinoma. J Clin Endocrinol Metab. 1990;71:414–24.
58. Shah JP, Loree TR, Dharker D, et al. Prognostic factors in differentiated carcinoma of the thyroid gland. Am J Surg. 1992;164:658–61.
59. Rossi RL, Cady B, Silverman MF, et al. Current results of conservative surgery for differentiated thyroid carcinoma. World J Surg. 1986;10:612–22.
60. Tisell LE, Nilsson B, Mölne J, et al. Improved survival of patients with papillary thyroid cancer after surgical microdissection. World J Surg. 1996;20:854–9.
61. Sellers M, Beenken S, Blankenship A, et al. Prognostic significance of cervical lymph node metastases in differentiated thyroid cancer. Am J Surg. 1992;164:578–81.
62. Hughes CJ, Shaha AR, Shah JP, et al. Impact of lymph node metastasis in differentiated carcinoma of the thyroid: a matched-pair analysis. Head Neck. 1996;18:127–32.

63. Lundgren CI, Hall P, Dickman PW, et al. Clinically significant prognostic factors for differentiated thyroid carcinoma: a population-based, nested case–control study. Cancer. 2006;106:524–31.
64. Shaha AR, Shah JP, Loree TR. Patterns of failure in differentiated carcinoma of the thyroid based on risk groups. Head Neck. 1998;20:26–30.
65. Harwood J, Clark OH, Dunphy JE. Significance of lymph node metastasis in differentiated thyroid cancer. Am J Surg. 1978;136:107–12.
66. Sugatini I, Yanagisawa A, Shimizu A, et al. Clinicopathologic and immunohistochemical studies of papillary thyroid microcarcinoma presenting with cervical lymphadenopathy. World J Surg. 1998;22:731–7.
67. Kitajiri S, Hiraumi H, Hirose T, et al. The presence of large lymph nodes metastasis as a prognostic factor of papillary thyroid carcinoma. Auris Nasus Larynx. 2003;30:169–74.
68. Ito Y, Fukushima M, Tomada C, et al. Prognosis of patients with papillary thyroid carcinoma having clinically apparent metastases to the lateral compartment. Endocr J. 2009;56:759–76.
69. Simpson WJ, McKinney SE, Carruthers JS, et al. Papillary and follicular thyroid cancer. Prognostic factors in 1,578 patients. Am J Med. 1987;83:479–88.
70. Leboulleux S, Rubino C, Baudin E, et al. Prognostic factors for persistent or recurrent disease of papillary thyroid carcinoma with neck lymph node metastases and/or tumor extension beyond the thyroid capsule at initial diagnosis. J Clin Endocrinol Metab. 2005;10:5723–9.
71. Beasley NJP, Lee J, Eski S, et al. Impact of nodal metastases on prognosis in patients with well-differentiated thyroid cancer. Arch Otolaryngol Head Neck Surg. 2002;128:825–8.
72. Randolph GW, Duh QY, Heller KS, et al. The prognostic significance of nodal metastases from papillary thyroid carcinoma can be stratified based on the size and number of metastatic lymph nodes, as well as the presence of extranodal extension. Thyroid. 2012;22:1144–52.
73. Ito Y, Higashiyama T, Takamura Y, et al. Risk factors for recurrence to the lymph node in papillary thyroid carcinoma patients without preoperatively detectable lateral node metastases: validity of prophylactic modified radical neck dissection. World J Surg. 2007;31:2085–91.
74. Ricarte-Filho J, Ganly I, Rivera M, et al. Papillary thyroid carcinomas with cervical lymph node metastases can be stratified into clinically relevant prognostic categories using oncogenic BRAF, the number of nodal metastases, and extra-nodal extension. Thyroid. 2012;22:575–84.
75. Sobin L, Gospodarowicz M, Wittekind C, editors. TNM classification of malignant tumors, Union for International Cancer Control. 7th ed. New York: Wiley-Blackwell; 2010.
76. Lim Y, Choi E, Yoon Y. Occult lymph nodes in neck level V in papillary thyroid carcinoma. Surgery. 2010;147:241–5.
77. Nam IC, Park JO, Joo YH, et al. Pattern and predictive factors of regional lymph node metastasis in papillary thyroid carcinoma: a prospective study. Head Neck. 2013;35:40–5.

Management of the Central Compartment in Well-Differentiated Thyroid Carcinoma

3

K. Alok Pathak, Rehan Kazi, and Richard W. Nason

Introduction

The central compartment of the neck is bounded superiorly by the hyoid bone, laterally by the carotid arteries, anteriorly by the superficial layer of the deep cervical fascia, posteriorly by the deep layer of the deep cervical fascia, and inferiorly by the innominate artery on the right and the corresponding axial plane on the left. [1] As illustrated in Fig. 3.1, the first echelon of lymphatic drainage of the thyroid is to the pretracheal, paratracheal and recurrent laryngeal nodes in the central compartment (level VI). This puts them at the highest risk of lymphatic metastasis in thyroid cancer. Subsequent lymphatic spread takes place to the superior mediastinal lymph nodes (level VII) and/or the lateral compartment of the neck (levels II–V), as has been outlined in Chap. 2 on lymph node metastasis in well-differentiated thyroid carcinoma (WDTC). Microscopic involvement of regional node occurs in 30–90 % of cases of papillary thyroid carcinomas (PTCs), with an incidence of clinically evident lymph node metastases at presentation ranging from 30 to 40 % [2–5]. The most commonly involved central lymph nodes in thyroid carcinoma are the prelaryngeal (Delphian), pretracheal, and the right and left paratracheal nodes [1].

K.A. Pathak (✉)
Head and Neck Surgical Oncology, CancerCare Manitoba, University of Manitoba,
675 McDermott Ave, Winnipeg, MB R3E0V9, Canada
e-mail: alok.pathak@cancercare.mb.ca

R. Kazi
Manipal University Karnataka, Manipal, India
e-mail: drrehankazi@gmail.com

R.W. Nason
Head and Neck Surgical Oncology, CancerCare Manitoba,
675 McDermott Ave, Winnipeg, MB R3E0V9, Canada
e-mail: nasonrw@cc.umanitoba.ca

© K. Alok Pathak, Richard W. Nason, Janice L. Pasieka, Rehan Kazi,
Raghav C. Dwivedi 2015
Springer India/Byword Books
K.A. Pathak et al. (eds.), *Management of Thyroid Cancer: Special Considerations*,
Head and Neck Cancer Clinics, DOI 10.1007/978-81-322-2434-1_3

Fig. 3.1 Levels VI and VII
lymph nodes in the central
compartment of the neck

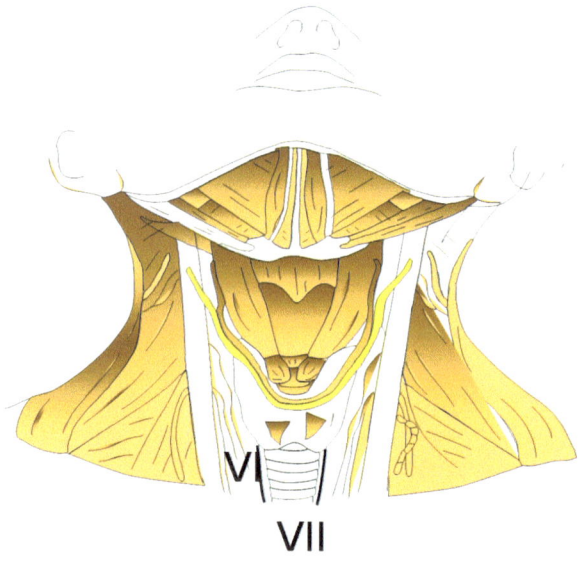

Fig. 3.2 Extent of central
compartment lymph node
dissection (*yellow area*)

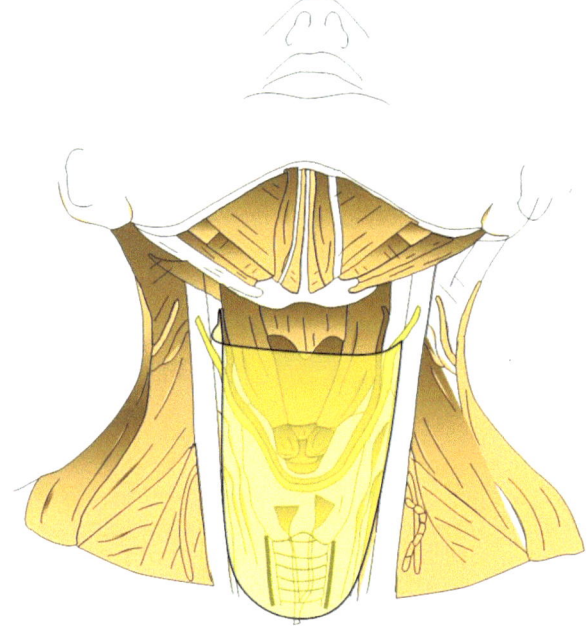

Central Compartment Neck Dissection

Central compartment lymph node dissection (Fig. 3.2) includes removal of the pretracheal and the paratracheal lymph nodes from the cricoid cartilage to the innominate artery on the right, and on the left to the axial plane where the innominate
crosses the trachea, along with the prelaryngeal lymph nodes [1]. It may be extended

to include additional nodal basins, such as the retropharyngeal, retro-oesophageal, paralaryngopharyngeal or superior mediastinal nodes. Removal of only the clinically involved nodes by 'plucking' or 'berry picking' of grossly involved lymph nodes rather than a complete nodal group removal may be associated with higher recurrence rates and morbidity from revision surgery [6]. Management of central compartment recurrence has been discussed further in Chap. 5 of this volume.

Central neck dissection can be either unilateral or bilateral and can be done either therapeutically or electively. A therapeutic central compartment neck dissection is performed when the nodal metastasis is clinically apparent (clinically N1a), whereas an elective central compartment dissection is prophylactic for nodal metastasis that is not detected clinically or radiologically (clinically N0). That a formal lymph node dissection should be performed in the setting of radiologically detected, biopsy-proven or palpable nodal disease is indisputable; however, its indication in the absence of discernible nodal disease, either in the central or lateral compartment of the neck, remains controversial. The American Thyroid Association (ATA) Guidelines Taskforce statement (2006) that routine central compartment (level VI) neck dissection should be considered for patients with PTC and suspected Hürthle cell carcinoma added to the controversy, both because of its ambiguity that led to vastly different interpretations among clinicians, and the paucity of strong data supporting it [7]. Thus, the revised guidelines (2009) state that prophylactic central compartment neck dissection (ipsilateral or bilateral) may be performed in patients with PTC with clinically uninvolved central neck lymph nodes, especially for advanced primary tumours (T3 or T4; grade C recommendation; expert opinion) [6]. A randomized controlled trial to answer this question is not considered feasible as it requires about 5,840 patients and over $20,000,000 [8].

Elective Central Neck Dissection

Evidence in Favour

Proponents for elective neck dissection argue that it can be completed with a low incidence of complications and reoperation in the central compartment, for recurrence is associated with a higher incidence of complications. Evidence supporting prophylactic neck dissection of the central compartment has been extrapolated from experience with medullary thyroid carcinoma (MTC). Tisell et al. developed the technique for microdissection for thyroid cancer using magnifying loops and bipolar cautery [9]. Dralle et al. described compartment-orientated microdissection for MTC with a low frequency of complications with respect to recurrent nerve injury and hypoparathyroidism (3.1 %) [10]. On the basis of these observations, the technique was extrapolated to patients of WDTC. Tisell's group reported on 195 patients with WDTC treated with total thyroidectomy and central node dissection [11]. The results were compared with contemporary series in other Scandinavian populations, including Norway and Finland. Death caused by thyroid cancer in their series was 1.6 % versus 8.4 % and 11.1 %, respectively, in the comparison groups. Scheumann et al. reported on 342 patients without making specific comparison between therapeutic versus elective neck dissection [12]. These authors stressed that for a tumour confined to the thyroid (no extrathyroidal extension), survival was increased by systematic compartment-orientated dissection. Sywak and co-workers showed the thyroglobulin levels to be lower in the group of 56 patients undergoing total thyroidectomy and central node dissection compared with 391 patients with total thyroidectomy alone [13]. The groups were comparable in terms of MACIS scores and radioactive iodine treatment. An undetectable thyroglobulin level was more likely with a central node dissection [13]. Total thyroidectomy resulted in 0.5 % hypoparathyroidism with no nerve injury, whereas for total thyroidectomy and ipsilateral central node dissection the rates were 1.8 % and 1.0 %, respectively. Gemsenjäger et al. noted hypocalcaemia in 2.4 % and recurrent nerve injury in 7.1 % of 42 patients undergoing therapeutic node dissections [14]. No hypocalcaemia or nerve injury was noted in the central node dissection or prophylactic node dissection group.

Evidence Against

Many surgeons feel that a prophylactic neck dissection is not indicated, as the nodal metastases can be removed when they become clinically evident in the majority of patients, and that the survival rates of patients treated prophylactically and therapeutically are comparable. The other argument against routine central node dissection is the widespread use of radioactive iodine, which may obscure the benefits of neck dissection. Whereas the results from Tisell's group were excellent, over a quarter of their patients had T1 disease [11]. It is not clear whether these patients would have done just as well with total thyroidectomy alone and no central neck dissection. Assessing the risk : benefit ratio of prophylactic neck dissections, Henry et al. evaluated complications after 50 total thyroidectomies for benign disease, and compared them to those in 50 patients with PTC (cN0) who were treated with total thyroidectomy and central node dissection [15]. The first group had three cases of transient nerve palsy (6 %) and 2 (4 %) in the second group. The multinodular group had no cases of permanent hypothyroidism, but 4 of transient hypoparathyroidism (8 %). In the thyroid cancer group, 7 patients developed transient hypoparathyroidism (14 %) and 2 patients (4 %) remained with definitive or permanent hypoparathyroidism. The authors concluded that after total thyroidectomy for PTC, central node dissection did not increase recurrent laryngeal nerve morbidity, but was responsible for a high rate of hypoparathyroidism, especially in the early postoperative course. They were of the opinion that even after taking into account the possible benefits, it is difficult to advocate routine central node dissection [15].

Roh et al. did not use a microdissection technique and reported hypocalcaemia in 30.5 % of patients after central compartment lymph node dissection [16]. In total thyroidectomy-alone group, the incidence of hypocalcaemia was 9.6 %. The mean number of parathyroid glands was 1.2 and was similar in the two groups. Four recurrences were observed: 3 of 73 of the total thyroidectomy alone, and 1 of 82 in the node dissection group. The central nodal group was involved in 62.2 % and the lateral group in 25.6 % recurrences. Considering overall survival, recurrence patterns and morbidity, these workers could not recommend routine use of central node dissection.

Pereira et al. reported a 60 % prevalence of positive lymphadenopathy in 43 clinically node-negative patients undergoing central node dissection and 58.1 % patients developed transient hypocalcaemia that was associated with incidental parathyroidectomy, number of nodes removed and thymectomy [17]. Permanent hypoparathyroidism was observed in 4.6 % of patients and transient vocal cord paralysis in 7 %. Central neck recurrences were not seen in any patient, but 5/43 patients developed lateral recurrences.

Frasoldati et al. described a series of patients in which there was no emphasis on central node dissection [18]. Central neck recurrence was observed in 5.8 % and it represented 60 % of all neck recurrences at 44 months, despite the use of radioactive iodine. Although central compartment node dissection is thought to reduce the risk of central neck failure, the same cannot be claimed about the lateral neck recurrences. This technique is also associated with a higher complication rate, especially of hypoparathyroidism.

Morbidity of Central Compartment Dissection

The morbidity from central compartment reoperation has been emphasized by several authors. Simon and colleagues studied 252 patients with WDTC; 77 patients had regionally recurrent thyroid cancer and underwent a reoperation [19]. The incidence of recurrent laryngeal nerve palsy or hypoparathyroidism was not significantly higher in post-recurrence surgery compared with the primary surgery. Similar finding were also observed by others during reoperation for recurrence [20, 21]. Cheah et al. described transient hypocalcaemia (defined as calcium of <2.0 mmol/L) in 23 % of patients undergoing 115 neck dissections, which was unrelated to the pathology, reoperation or extent of lymphadenectomy [22]. Kupferman et al. reported 21 % transient hypocalcaemia, no permanent hypocalcaemia, and two transient recurrent nerve paresis in 33 central neck dissections [23]. Kim et al. described morbidities after central neck reoperations [24]. They used recurrent laryngeal nerve monitoring with a wire placed in the vocal cord; recurrent nerve paralysis was not seen, 20 % of patients had transient hypocalcaemia, and 5 % had permanent hypoparathyroidism. These authors concluded that with meticulous dissection and neurological monitoring, a reoperation can be done safely.

It is true that elective central compartment lymph node dissection may upstage some patients from clinical N0 to pathological N1a; its influence on reducing the central compartment recurrence rates does not translate into improved survival. This advantage needs to be balanced against a higher morbidity, primarily recurrent laryngeal nerve injury and transient hypoparathyroidism, with questionable oncological benefit [16, 25, 26].

Consensus on Management of Central Compartment Lymph Nodes

The ATA guidelines recommend a therapeutic central compartment (level VI) neck dissection for patients with clinically involved central or lateral neck lymph nodes, in addition to total thyroidectomy [6]. For small (T1 or T2), non-invasive, clinically node-negative PTCs and most FTCs, a neartotal or total thyroidectomy without prophylactic central neck dissection might be appropriate and a prophylactic central-compartment neck dissection (ipsilateral or bilateral) may be performed in patients with PTC with clinically uninvolved central neck lymph nodes, especially for advanced primary tumours (T3 or T4). However, caution should be exercised when interpreting these recommendations in view of available surgical expertise. For patients with small, non-invasive, apparently node-negative tumours, the balance of risk and benefit may favour simple near-total thyroidectomy with close intraoperative inspection of the central compartment with compartmental dissection, only in the presence of obviously involved lymph nodes. This approach may increase the chance of future locoregional recurrence, but overall this approach may be safer in less experienced surgical hands.

The authors' Approach to the Central Compartment

The authors believe in a conservative approach that 'an operation not worth doing is not worth doing well'. We routinely assess the ipsilateral central compartment at the time of thyroidectomy for WDTCs. Any suspicious node, which is either visible or palpable in the central compartment, is sent for frozen section. If nodal metastasis is confirmed, a therapeutic dissection is undertaken. Multiple lymph nodes necessitate a bilateral central compartment lymph node dissection. In the presence of lateral neck metastasis with an uninvolved central neck, an ipsilateral central compartment lymph node dissection is undertaken.

While performing total thyroidectomy, the recurrent laryngeal nerves and parathyroid glands are identified. Utmost care is taken to preserve the parathyroid glands on the less involved sides, along with its blood supply from the inferior thyroid artery. The recurrent laryngeal nerve needs to be exposed throughout its course in the central compartment of the neck with minimal manipulation of the nerve. The entire lympho-areolar tissue in the central compartment is excised, extending from the carotid sheath laterally to the tracheo-oesophageal groove medially (Figs 3.2 and 3.3) and extending from the level of the thyroid cartilage superiorly to the level of the innominate artery in the superior mediastinum inferiorly. Grossly involved nodes identified in the mediastinum tend to be in continuity and are bound together with adipose and areolar tissue, which facilitates delivery of the nodes through the cervical approach. Extensive metastases to more inferior locations in the mediastinum, which are not accessible to the cervical incision, are uncommon and rarely require a sternotomy. Our team makes every effort to identify and preserve at least two normal, vascularized parathyroid glands. If a parathyroid gland is inadvertently

Fig. 3.3 Intraoperative photograph of the right central compartment lymph node dissection showing the right common carotid artery (*CCA*) laterally and trachea medially. Right recurrent laryngeal nerve (*Rt. RLN*) and right superior and inferior parathyroid glands (*white arrows*) have been identified

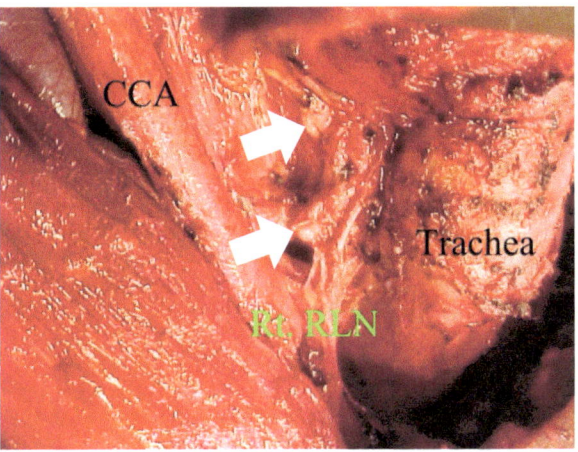

removed or devascularized, it is auto-transplantated into a muscular pocket in the sternocleidomastoid muscle, after frozen section confirmation of a small sample of parathyroid tissue to reduce the risk of tumour transplantation. The pocket is closed and identified by 3-0 non-absorbable suture. Intraoperative nerve monitoring (IONM) is not used routinely.

Use of IONM is another area of debate. The routine use of IONM varies, depending on the training, surgical experience and practice set-up; however, it is not an alternative for proper identification and meticulous dissection of the nerve. Even in the USA the use of IONM varies considerably from the community to the university hospitals and from one specialty to another [27, 28]. Dralle et al. in their review, comparing IONM to visual examination, did not find any statistically significant difference in the recurrent laryngeal nerve paralysis in the two groups [29]. Negative predictive values were high (NPV 92–100 %), but relatively low and variable positive predictive values (PPV 10–90 %) for IONM, which limited its utility for intraoperative right laryngeal nerve management.

To summarize, even though a routine central compartment microdissection for differentiated carcinoma of the thyroid can be performed safely, with excellent results by the surgeons who are skilled and experienced in the technique, it is unlikely that such excellent results would be achieved by less experienced surgeons. As evidence to indicate superior oncological results in the clinically N0 neck with this approach is unclear, to minimize the resulting morbidity, a prophylactic central compartment lymph node dissection should be used judiciously and based on the aggressiveness of the disease and available surgical expertise.

References

1. American Thyroid Association Surgery Working Group, American Association of Endocrine Surgeons, American Academy of Otolaryngology-Head and Neck Surgery, American Head and Neck Society, Carty SE, Cooper DS, Doherty GM, et al. Consensus statement on the ter-

minology and classification of central neck dissection for thyroid cancer. Thyroid. 2009;19:1153–8.

2. White ML, Gauger PG, Doherty GM. Central lymph node dissection in differentiated thyroid cancer. World J Surg. 2007;31:895–904.

3. Mazzaferri EL, Young RL. Papillary thyroid carcinoma: a 10 year follow-up report of the impact of therapy in 576 patients. Am J Med. 1981;70:511–8.

4. Sanders LE, Rossi RL. Occult well differentiated thyroid carcinoma presenting as cervical node disease. World J Surg. 1995;19:642–7.

5. Cady B, Sedgwick CE, Meissner WA, et al. Changing clinical, pathologic, therapeutic, and survival patterns in differentiated thyroid carcinoma. Ann Surg. 1976;184:541–53.

6. American Thyroid Association (ATA) Guidelines Taskforce on Thyroid Nodules and Differentiated Thyroid Cancer, Cooper DS, Doherty GM, Haugen BR, et al. Revised American Thyroid Association management guidelines for patients with thyroid nodules and differentiated thyroid cancer. Thyroid. 2009;19:1167–214.

7. Cooper DS, Doherty GM, Haugen BR, et al.; American Thyroid Association Guidelines Taskforce. Management guidelines for patients with thyroid nodules and differentiated thyroid cancer. Thyroid. 2006;16:109–42.

8. Carling T, Carty SE, Ciarleglio MM, et al.; American Thyroid Association Surgical Affairs Committee. American Thyroid Association design and feasibility of a prospective randomized controlled trial of prophylactic central lymph node dissection for papillary thyroid carcinoma. Thyroid. 2012;22:237–44.

9. Tisell LE, Hansson G, Jansson S, et al. Reoperation in the treatment of asymptomatic metastasizing medullary thyroid carcinoma. Surgery. 1986;99:60–6.

10. Dralle H, Damm I, Scheumann GF, et al. Frequency and significance of cervicomediastinal lymph node metastases in medullary thyroid carcinoma: results of a compartment-oriented microdissection method. Henry Ford Hosp Med J. 1992;40:264–7.

11. Tisell LE, Nilsson B, Mölne J, et al. Improved survival of patients with papillary thyroid cancer after surgical microdissection. World J Surg. 1996;20:854–9.

12. Scheumann GF, Grimm O, Wegener G, et al. Prognostic significance and surgical management of locoregional lymph node metastases in papillary thyroid cancer. World J Surg. 1994;18:559–67; discussion 567–8.

13. Sywak M, Cornford L, Roach P, et al. Routine ipsilateral level VI lymphadenectomy reduces postoperative thyroglobulin levels in papillary thyroid cancer. Surgery. 2006;140:1000–5; discussion 1005–7.

14. Gemsenjäger E, Perren A, Seifert B, et al. Lymph node surgery in papillary thyroid carcinoma. J Am Coll Surg. 2003;197:182–90.

15. Henry JF, Gramatica L, Denizot A, et al. Morbidity of prophylactic lymph node dissection in the central neck area in patients with papillary thyroid carcinoma. Langenbecks Arch Surg. 1998;383:167–9.

16. Roh JL, Park JY, Park CI. Total thyroidectomy plus neck dissection in differentiated papillary thyroid carcinoma patients: pattern of nodal metastasis, morbidity, recurrence, and postoperative levels of serum parathyroid hormone. Ann Surg. 2007;245:604–10.

17. Pereira JA, Jimeno J, Miquel J, et al. Nodal yield, morbidity, and recurrence after central neck dissection for papillary thyroid carcinoma. Surgery. 2005;138:1095–100.

18. Frasoldati A, Pesenti M, Gallo M, et al. Diagnosis of neck recurrences in patients with differentiated thyroid carcinoma. Cancer. 2003;97:90–6.

19. Simon D, Goretzki PE, Witte J, et al. Incidence of regional recurrence guiding radicality in differentiated thyroid carcinoma. World J Surg. 1996;20:860–6.

20. Segal K, Friedental R, Lubin E, et al. Papillary carcinoma of the thyroid. Otolaryngol Head Neck Surg. 1995;113:356–63.

21. Alvarado R, Sywak MS, Delbridge L, et al. Central lymph node dissection as a secondary procedure for papillary thyroid cancer: Is there added morbidity? Surgery. 2009;145:514–8.

22. Cheah WK, Arici C, Ituarte PH, et al. Complications of neck dissection for thyroid cancer. World J Surg. 2002;26:1013–6.
23. Kupferman ME, Patterson DM, Mandel SJ, et al. Safety of modified radical neck dissection for differentiated thyroid carcinoma. Laryngoscope. 2004;114:403–6.
24. Kim ES, Kim TY, Koh JM, et al. Completion thyroidectomy in patients with thyroid cancer who initially underwent unilateral operation. Clin Endocrinol (Oxf). 2004;61:145–8.
25. Moley JF, Wells SA. Compartment-mediated dissection for papillary thyroid cancer. Langenbecks Arch Surg. 1999;384:9–15.
26. Cavicchi O, Piccin O, Caliceti U, et al. Transient hypoparathyroidism following thyroidectomy: a prospective study and multivariate analysis of 604 consecutive patients. Otolaryngol Head Neck Surg. 2007;137:654–8.
27. Horne SK, Gal TJ, Brennan JA. Prevalence and patterns of intraoperative nerve monitoring for thyroidectomy. Otolaryngol Head Neck Surg. 2007;136:952–6.
28. Sturgeon C, Sturgeon T, Angelos P. Neuromonitoring in thyroid surgery: attitudes, usage patterns, and predictors of use among endocrine surgeons. World J Surg. 2009;33:417–25.
29. Dralle H, Sekulla C, Lorenz K, et al. ; German IONM Study Group. Intraoperative monitoring of the recurrent laryngeal nerve in thyroid surgery. World J Surg. 2008;32:1358–66.

Management of the Lateral Neck in Well-Differentiated Thyroid Cancer

4

Richard W. Nason and K. Alok Pathak

Introduction

Lymph node metastases to the lateral neck in well-differentiated thyroid cancer (WDTC) do not appear to significantly impact overall survival. They probably do play a role in recurrence- and disease-free survival. As reviewed elsewhere in this monograph the extent of surgical resection should depend on the extent of cancer with the aim to control the cancer and avoid reoperation if possible with minimal morbidity. Management decisions for the lateral neck are based on desire for regional control balanced with complications of surgery. These considerations have driven controversy in both the timing of treatment (elective versus therapeutic neck dissection) and the extent of surgery necessary to control disease. At present, the balance of opinion favours observation or expectant management of the clinically negative lateral neck. The extent of neck dissection for clinically evident disease remains controversial.

R.W. Nason (✉)
Head and Neck Surgical Oncology, CancerCare Manitoba,
675 McDermott Ave, Winnipeg, MB R3E0V9, Canada
e-mail: nasonrw@cc.umanitoba.ca

K.A. Pathak
Head and Neck Surgical Oncology, CancerCare Manitoba, University of Manitoba,
675 McDermott Ave, Winnipeg, MB R3E0V9, Canada
e-mail: alok.pathak@cancercare.mb.ca

© K. Alok Pathak, Richard W. Nason, Janice L. Pasieka, Rehan Kazi, 39
Raghav C. Dwivedi 2015
Springer India/Byword Books
K.A. Pathak et al. (eds.), *Management of Thyroid Cancer: Special Considerations*,
Head and Neck Cancer Clinics, DOI 10.1007/978-81-322-2434-1_4

Timing of Neck Dissection

Elective treatment of the lateral neck has received strong support. Prophylactic neck dissection has been favoured in Japan [1, 2]. Noguchi and Murakami cited low recurrence rates in patients treated with modified radical neck dissection, with more survivors in the >40-year age group [1]. These surgeons routinely performed a modified radical neck dissection in patients >40-year-old with tumours larger than 1.5 cm. In assessing the results of an international survey, Noguchi and Murakami [1] concluded that ipsilateral modified neck dissection might be justified in all patients, including those with 'minimal thyroid cancer', arguing that this procedure reduced lymph node recurrence and avoided the need for reoperation. They also advocated bilateral modified neck dissection with involvement of bilateral lobes cancer in the isthmus, or contralateral or bilateral palpable nodes. Because of the significance of the central nodes, they stressed the importance of a careful dissection to avoid morbidity. These authors commented on the significance of the central nodes and the importance of a careful dissection in this area to avoid morbidity. In contrast they said that lateral jugular lymph nodes rarely affect life expectancy and that dissection of the lateral nodes can be performed with minimal additional morbidity.

In 1990, Noguchi and co-workers published results of a multivariate analysis on 218 patients with WDTC [3]. They noted that before 1972 most patients were managed conservatively with 'node picking' for palpable disease. From 1973 onward, most patients underwent a modified radical neck dissection. After controlling for the effect of confounding variables in this series (viz. age, sex and extended thyroidectomy), survival was greater in the group managed with elective neck dissection as a component of treatment. In 80 cases treated before 1972, regional recurrence rate was 15.9 %, with an overall survival of 89 %. Twenty-four patients from this group underwent a 'node picking procedure' for palpable disease. One hundred and thirty-two patients comprised the group treated from 1973 to 1983. These patients were treated with subtotal thyroidectomy and modified radical neck dissection, which was prophylactic in 101 patients. The recurrence rate in the lymph nodes was 7 % and overall survival was 97 %. The relative risk of death with the conservative approach was 17.3 (p < 0.005). In this series, radioactive iodine was not used. All patients did, however, receive suppressive doses of thyroid hormone. It is to be noted that the presence of both clinical and histological lymph node involvement was not identified as unfavourable prognostic factors.

Elective treatment of the neck has received support in North America as well. Attie et al. supported the use of this procedure citing the high incidence of nodal metastases, and noting results of several retrospective reviews where recurrences in cervical nodes and subsequent death were emphasized [4]. Frankenthaler and co-workers studied 117 patients <20 years of age with who were treated at MD Anderson [5]. A high incidence of recurrences was seen (29 %, of which 24 % were in the neck) [5]. To maintain a low rate of recurrence (there were no deaths in this series), these authors recommended near-total thyroidectomy with modified neck dissection followed by ^{131}I treatment. They argued that neck dissections are associated with a low incidence of complications. After completing 800 conservative neck dissections, Noguchi and Murakami reported that injury to the spinal accessory nerve occurred in 1 % of patients, Horner syndrome in 0.5 %, lymphatic fistula in 0.1 %, and hypoglossal nerve injury in 0.1 % [1].

The balance of opinion currently favours therapeutic neck dissection in the presence of biopsy-proven disease. There is no prospective randomized data to explore the impact of elective node dissection on recurrence or disease-specific mortality in papillary thyroid cancer [6, 7]. Clinical observations suggest that nodal metastases may be removed when they become clinically evident in the majority of patients and that the survival of patients treated prophylactically and therapeutically are comparable [8–12]. In reviewing 1,079 patients treated at Memorial Sloan-Kettering (USA) from 1930 to 1959, Hutter estimated that eight neck dissections would have to be done to prevent the later appearance of cervical node metastases in one patient who would probably be cured by therapeutic dissection when the neck recurrence was identified [12]. Although it is known that metastases are frequent, it is apparent that most do not achieve clinical significance. The incidence of clinical recurrence in the neck in patients who do not undergo nodal excision has been recognized to be low, ~7–15 % [1, 13, 14]. Cady and Rossi observed that most low-risk patients with neck recurrences are managed successfully [11].

A study by Hamming and co-workers from the Netherlands Cancer Institute is cited frequently in support of treatment of positive nodes only [10]. They compared 84 patients treated with total thyroidectomy and resection of positive lymph nodes only, with 81 patients treated with total thyroidectomy, routine dissection of the trachea-oesophageal groove, frozen sections of lymph nodes from the internal jugular vein, and if metastases were found, a modified neck dissection on the affected side. The two groups were comparable in age, sex and stage. Almost twice as many patients were found to have metastases in the neck dissection group. No significant difference was seen in 10-year overall or recurrence-free survival between the two groups. The neck dissection group had more instances of hypoparathyroidism and accessory nerve palsies ($p < 0.05$). Thus, when a more extensive search for metastases was conducted, more metastases of cervical lymph nodes were detected, but this did not prevent recurrence in the neck nor did it improve survival time. This approach resulted in more postoperative morbidity. These authors concluded that prophylactic removal of regional lymph nodes in instances of PTC is unjustified. Shah et al. reported on 74 patients with WDTC who underwent a neck dissection in a Toronto hospital [15]. Central node dissection was performed in 6 patients, lateral neck dissection in 47, and central and lateral neck dissection in 21. The recurrence rates in these three groups in the central and lateral compartments, and the incidence of distant recurrence were similar ($p > 0.05$). They recommended dissection of only the central and lateral compartments in the presence of positive disease. Gemsenjäger et al. studied 159 unselected patients who were followed for 1–27 years [16]. Forty-two N1 (pN1 98 %) underwent a therapeutic lymphadenectomy, 29 N0 (pN1 17 %) underwent a prophylactic neck dissection, and 88 N0 (pN1 2.3 %) were merely observed. The review, spanning from 1974 to 2000, showed that lymphadenectomy was used more frequently in the latter years of the study. This led to a non-significant increase in pN1 stage (stage migration)—from 26 to 30 %. Neck recurrences were identified in 12 % of the pN1 and 3 % of the pN0 patients. They were distributed equally between the central and lateral compartments. Wada et al. evaluated lymph node metastases in 259 patients with WDTC [17]. Twenty-four patients had palpable nodes and underwent a therapeutic neck dissection. Two hundred and thirty-five underwent an elective or prophylactic neck dissection. The incidence of lymph node involvement in the central compartment was 64.1 % and lateral compartment was 44.5 %. Neck recurrence was 0.43 % after elective neck dissection, 0.65 % with no dissection, and 16.7 % in the therapeutic group.

Proponents of therapeutic neck dissections note that shoulder disability is significant even without dividing the spinal accessory nerve. Temporary or permanent weakness occurs in as many as 20 % of patients [18]. In summary, elective dissection of the lateral compartment of the neck is not supported. It is agreed that morbidity does not increase with treatment of metachronous disease in this compartment.

Extent of Dissection

The consensus is to treat only clinically positive lymph nodes in the lateral neck. The extent of dissection continues to generate controversy. Before 1960, the standard radical neck dissection was not infrequently used in managing the neck in WDTC [4, 19–21]. Sanders and Rossi [22] in their review of 92 patients presenting with a lateral neck mass noted that before 1960 a standard radical neck dissection was used in 84 % of patients. George Crile Jr was among the first and most vocal opponents of the routine use of the standard radical neck dissection in treating WDTC [20]. His arguments centred on the overall good prognosis of patients with WDTC. He presented anatomical evidence that it was not possible to apply the en bloc principle or to excise the primary cancer in continuity with its metastases. For example, he noted that the thyroid lies in a fascial compartment of its own that has no continuity with the lateral cervical region and is separated from it by the carotid vessels, which cannot be sacrificed. He emphasized the importance of the central zone. Death did not occur from uncontrollable PTC in the lateral cervical region; it comes from central recurrences of the primary tumour or its metastases. The battle of the thyroid was won or lost in the central area of the mediastinum or neck and it is this critical area that the classical radical neck dissection disregards. In citing his experience with modified neck dissection in 73 patients, 64 % had metastases and none died of cancer or developed distant metastases. The modification, he emphasized, was preservation of the sternocleidomastoid. He described its removal as mutilating, particularly in a population of patients that tended to be young. He felt that the conventional bloc dissection when applied to cancer of the thyroid should be abandoned.

Others refined and supported the technique of modified radical neck dissection as applied to thyroid cancer and confirmed a high degree of reasonable control with the procedure [4, 19]. Marchetta et al. stressed the importance of sparing the accessory nerve [19]. Their procedure also preserved the internal jugular vein. These authors divided the sternocleidomastoid to facilitate this dissection. Attie et al. did not divide the sternocleidomastoid muscle, noting that transection and re-suturing often led to atrophy and contracture [4]. It was routine for them to sacrifice the internal jugular vein in unilateral dissections. The balance of opinion was that a modified radical neck dissection with preservation of the accessory nerve, sterno-cleidomastoid, and internal jugular vein was equally effective as a radical neck dissection when applied to PTC.

Subsequently, more limited neck dissections, the node or 'berry picking' procedures, were favoured. Crile, in 1950 [23], was among the earliest to perform more limited surgery with 'enucleation or picking out' of individual nodes. This practice received support in Mazzaferri and Young's retrospective review in 1981 [24]. Patients undergoing more extensive neck dissections had more complications and no survival benefit. Major postoperative complications were observed in >40 % of patients treated with total thyroidectomy combined with extensive neck dissection; in contrast, when total thyroidectomy was combined with regional node excision, major complications occurred in only 13 % of patients [24]. A similar conclusion was reached in the previously cited study by Hamming and co-workers in which a greater amount of postoperative morbidity was found in patients undergoing more extensive surgery, with accessory nerve palsies reaching statistical significance ($p < 0.05$). These authors supported the use of limited neck dissections with minimal clinical involvement of cervical lymph nodes. Sanders and Rossi, in a review of 92 patients with thyroid cancer presenting as a lateral neck mass, noted no alteration in survival with a radical neck dissection (97.5 %), modified radical neck dissection (85.6 %), or limited dissection (100 %) [22].

It is currently recognized that the limited 'node' or 'berry picking' procedures are associated with an unacceptable level of recurrence. McGregor and co-workers found no difference between node picking and modified radical neck dissection when lymph nodes were only minimally involved (<5 nodes); however, with more extensive disease (>5 nodes) the ultimate rate of failure to control disease in the neck was felt to be unacceptably high among the patients who initially underwent conservative localized neck dissection [25]. In a retrospective review of anatomical neck dissections and 'berry picking' procedures, recurrence of 100 % was identified after a berry picking procedure versus 9 % after a more formal neck dissection ($p < 0.0001$) [26].

In a retrospective cohort study from 1958 to 2002, in which patients underwent primary thyroid surgery for PTC in a specialist centre in Italy. Palazzo et al. [27] reported that the percentage of patients who had a lymphadenectomy increased from 20 % in 1958 to 48 % in 2002, of which 84 % underwent a selective lymph node dissection. These workers noted that the trend towards more frequent use of neck dissection was most significant over the past 10 years. During this four and a half decade study, the initial trend was away from berry picking towards a modified radical neck dissection and, later, a trend away from this towards a selective neck dissection. The most common practice at present involves compartment-oriented and level-specific dissections. Evidence suggests that selective neck dissections achieve similar disease control to comprehensive neck dissections [28, 29]. The extent or type of selective neck dissection varies (Table 4.1).

Dissection of level I is unnecessary unless clinical evidence of disease supports it. It is universally agreed that dissection of levels III and IV is necessary. Most surgeons support dissection of level II. Grant and co-workers are of the opinion that

Table 4.1 Recommended levels of dissection for therapeutic neck dissections in WDTC

Series	Levels dissected
Sivanandan and Soo (2001) [37]	II–IV
Pingpank et al. (2002) [38]	II–V
Caron et al. (2006) [34]	III, IV
Yanir and Doweck (2008) [39]	II–V
Kupferman et al. (2008) [40]	II–V
Farrag et al. (2009) [31]	IIa, III, IV, Vb
Yuce et al. (2010) [41]	II–V
Grant et al. (2010) [30]	III, IV, Vb
Lim et al. (2010) [32]	II–IV
Ahmadi et al. (2011) [33]	II–IV

only a modest extension of the thyroidectomy incision is necessary to dissect levels III, IV and Va [30]. Treatment of level II requires a significantly larger incision and exposure. They express concern over the relatively high complication rates associated with more extensive neck dissections. Level II is addressed by these workers when clinical or radiological disease is evident. In their series of 420 patients studied over a 7-year period, Grant and co-workers identified a relapse in level II in only one patient [30]. In Farrag and associates' experience, level IIb is never involved in isolation and they only address the area above and lateral to the accessory nerve if level IIa is involved [31]. The prospect of shoulder dysfunction from the dissection of the accessory nerve has limited the dissection of level V by some investigators [30–33]. Ahmadi and co-workers noted that level V was never involved in isolation [33]. When treating level V they limit dissection in the posterior triangle to the area below the accessory nerve. The accessory nerve and its course in the posterior triangle are identified to avoid injury to the nerve; however, circumferential dissection is avoided. Lim et al. also emphasized that level V is not involved in isolation, and only in the presence of positive nodes in level IV [32]. They dissect level V only if histological evidence confirms involvement of level IV. Caron and co-workers target levels III and IV. Level II is addressed with extensive involvement of level III and level V is dissected only in the presence of clinical or radiological evidence of disease [34]. They have been able to achieve good disease control.

The Authors' Approach

Lymph nodes in the lateral neck in WDTC are treated with a selective neck dissection of levels IIa, III, IV and Vb, in keeping with current guidelines [35]. Histological confirmation is recommended before proceeding with a selective lateral neck dissection. In the experience of the present authors, most palpable nodes in patients with PTC are positive. In patients presenting primarily with lateral neck disease, the selective lateral neck dissection is done in conjunction with a total/near-total thyroidectomy and a central compartment dissection. When the lateral neck is treated remote from the initial thyroidectomy, addressing the central compartment is individualized to the patient. In this situation, judgement regarding reoperation in the central compartment involves reviewing the details of the initial operation, including the management of the paratracheal lymph nodes, the recurrent laryngeal nerve and the parathyroids. The functional status of the parathyroids and recurrent laryngeal nerve needs to be assessed. Careful attention is paid to the status of the central compartment with preoperative imaging, using both ultrasound and CT, and intraoperative assessment.

Technique

The procedure is performed under general anaesthesia without paralysis to facilitate identification of nerves. A nerve stimulator should be available. Exposure for this dissection can be achieved by extending the thyroidectomy incision laterally and superiorly at its posterior extent, if necessary. The use of a separate transverse incision superiorly (McFee incision) may facilitate exposure in the long neck and with the involvement of upper neck nodes. Skin flaps are elevated in the subplatysmal plane. It is important to consider that the platysma thins out in the posterior triangle and that the accessory nerve runs a superficial course. The anterior boarder of the trapezius is exposed. The accessory nerve (AN) is identified. One of the authors (R.W. Nason) uses the nerve point in the posterior triangle [36]. An imaginary line is drawn from the thyroid notch to the point at which the sensory nerve emerges from behind the posterior board of the sternocleidomastoid muscle (SCM). The midpoint of the SCM approximates this point. The AN enters the posterior triangle within 2 cm above this line, and exits posteriorly beneath the trapezius muscle within 2 cm below. A haemostat is used to spread dense fascia and areolar tissue along the posterior border of the SCM to identify the AN where it enters the posterior triangle. The course of the nerve is identified without circumferential dissection. The dissection is started inferiorly dividing the distal external jugular vein and transecting the lymphoareolar tissue between ties until the plane of dissection is established on the deep layer of cervical fascia. The lymphoareolar tissue below the course of the AN is mobilized from the anterior board of the trapezius and immediately on the posterior compartment muscles, which include the splenius capitis, levator scapulae and the scalene muscles. With dissection on the medial board of the levator scapulae, the cervical plexus is encountered. These cutaneous sensory branches are divided in the presence of bulky disease. With minimal node involvement they can be preserved. The phrenic nerve is identified on the surface of the anterior scalene muscle. The SCM is mobilized from the carotid sheath and retracted cephalad and medially. Medial retraction of the specimen exposes the internal jugular vein. The specimen is then mobilized from the vein with sharp dissection and subsequently from the carotid artery with attention to the course of the vagus nerve. The specimen is passed underneath the SCM and with the muscle retracted laterally and inferiorly the dissection of the carotid sheath is completed in the anterior triangle. The dissection of the upper carotid sheath is completed above the level of posterior belly of digastric. If it is necessary to continue superiorly to the skull base (level IIb dissection), the hypoglossal nerve is identified and followed superiorly to identify the proximal internal jugular vein and the accessory nerve in the anterior triangle before it enters the SCM [36]. It is generally not possible, or for that matter necessary, to maintain continuity between the resected thyroid and lymphoareolar contents of the central compartment and lateral compartment.

Commentary on Chaps. 2, 3 and 4

Janice L. Pasieka
What to do with the lymph nodes in well-differentiated thyroid cancer
Recently, the management of the lymph node compartments in well-differentiated thyroid cancer (WDTC) has been the focus of much debate among the surgeons and endocrinologists dealing with this disease. Why has there been so much recent 'press' on this topic? Much of this has to do with the changing paradigm in the definition of thyroid cancer recurrence. Until a decade ago the identification of recurrence in WDTC relied on physical examination and/or the demonstration of disease on follow-up radioactive I^{131} scans. This has changed with the advent of high-resolution ultra-sounds and the measurement of stimulated thyroglobulin (Tg) levels. These technological advances have allowed for the identification of disease that was too small to detect by physical examination and I^{131} scanning. As such, the definition of persistent and recurrent disease has changed in recent years. Because of this, endocrinologists, medical oncologists and surgeons have questioned whether more extensive surgical removal of the disease at the first operation would benefit this patient population—hence the development of prophylactic central neck dissections (pCLNDs).

In this monograph, Pathak and Nason have described their approaches to both the central and lateral neck compartments in WDTC. The American Thyroid Association (ATA) set out to provide guidance on the issue of pCLND, yet recognized early that uniformity in definitions was needed to interpret the current literature. Carty et al. defined the central neck and introduced definitions for ipsilateral and bilateral level VI dissections [1]. It is important that surgeons operating for thyroid cancer are familiar with these standardized definitions. Level VI includes the tissue between the carotid sheaths from the hyoid bone to the innominate artery. This includes the pyramidal lobe, forgotten by many, the anterior peritracheal tissue and the tissue deep in the neck in which the inferior parathyroid gland and recurrent laryngeal nerve (RLN) lie. It is because of the close proximity of the RLN to the parathyroid glands that pCLND should not be taken lightly [2, 3]. Although risk to the RLN appears to be similar to that from total thyroidectomy alone, hypoparathyroidism is increased, especially when bilateral pCLNDs are performed [2, 3]. The clinical benefit of removing clinically negative nodes (cN0) from this compartment has been discussed extensively in the literature. Most authors would agree that to date no survival benefit is seen in patients undergoing a pCLND for WDTC [4]. Some have argued that CLND decreases postoperative serum thyroglobulin (Tg) levels, thus decreasing recurrence/persistence rates [5]. The oncological principle of removing the draining lymph node basin for most cancers is to stage the patient accurately, and as such, influence postoperative therapy. Forty per cent of patients with cN0 disease were up-staged as a result of the histological findings on pCLND. Not surprising, given the high incidence of positive lymph nodes in WDTC. However, in centres that provide selective I^{131} ablative therapy, pCLND has led to an increased utilization of I^{131} therapy in 33 % of WDTC patients [6]. Many centres utilize a more selective use of I^{131} therapy in low-risk patients because of the lack of survival benefit seen with its use [7]. Thus, for the individual surgeon dealing with WDTC, the need for pCLND must be individualized to that surgeon and their referral cancer centre. First, the surgeon must know his/her rate of RLN injury and hypoparathyroidism with CLND. Second, the surgeon has to understand how the additional information from the central lymph nodes will be utilized. If their centre routinely gives I^{131} to all patients regardless of the risk status, then pCLND may be of little benefit. If the centre selectively gives therapy to all N1 disease, providing the additional staging information gained from the pCLND may be of some benefit. Yet clinically, most clinicians recognize that there are varying degrees of magnitude in the risk for recurrence for N1 disease. The upstaging of low-risk patients with small-volume nodal disease conveys a much smaller risk of recurrence than those with large-volume disease. Randolph et al. have recently proposed an N1 stratification for the use of I^{131} therapy [8]. Their document provides a rational approach to the question of how to utilize the information provided from a CLND.

A prospective, randomized controlled trial of pCLND in WDTC would help clarify this issue for the surgeons. However, given the low rates of both structural recurrence and morbidity after surgery for cN0 disease, prohibitively large sample sizes would be required for sufficient statistical power to demonstrate significant differences in outcomes [9]. Biochemical molecular tumour markers are gaining wider use in clinical practice and in time, hopefully, will provide more specific information on which surgical decision-making can be based [4, 10].

Clinically positive lymph nodes warrant a compartmental dissection, as outlined by Pathak and Nason in this monograph. The utilization of preoperative lymph node mapping with ultrasound has become the standard of care in most North American centres. Recent changes in the ATA guidelines for medullary thyroid cancer have moved from routine lateral neck dissections to selected dissections of the lateral compartments on the basis of lymph node mapping [11]. Although this approach relies on the sensitivity of thyroid ultrasonography, surgeons, endocrinologists, along with radiologists are becoming more skilled with this adjunct in the clinical evaluation of the thyroid and its regional lymph node basins. Most clinicians have expanded the role of ultrasound lymph node mapping with fine-needle aspiration confirmation to WDTC. This approach helps prepare both the patient and the surgeon preoperatively.

Lymph node metastases are common in WDTC. Clinically positive lymph nodes require a compartment dissection. The surgical approach to the regional nodal basin in cN0 disease is currently under debate. Risk versus benefit for the patient should continue to guide the surgeon when treating WDTC.

References

1. Carty SE, Cooper DS, Doherty GM, et al. Consensus statement on the terminology and classification of central neck dissection for thyroid cancer. Thyroid. 2009;19:1153–8.

2. Giordano D, Valcavi R, Thompson GB, et al. Complications of central neck dissection in patients with papillary thyroid carcinoma: results of a study on 1087 patients and review of the literature. Thyroid. 2012;22:911–17.

3. Paek SH, Lee YM, Min SY, et al. Risk factors of hypoparathyroidism following total thyroidectomy for thyroid cancer. World J Surg. 2013;37:94–101.

4. Yeung MJ, Pasieka JL. Well-differentiated thyroid carcinomas: management of the central lymph node compartment and emerging biochemical markers. J Oncol. 2011;2011:705305.

5. Sywak M, Cornford L, Roach P, et al. Routine ipsilateral level VI lymphadenectomy reduces postoperative thyroglobulin levels in papillary thyroid cancer. Surgery. 2006;140:1000–5; discussion 1005–7.

6. Wang TS, Evans DB, Fareau GG, et al. Effect of prophylactic central compartment neck dissection on serum thyroglobulin and recommendations for adjuvant radioactive iodine in patients with differentiated thyroid cancer. Ann Surg Oncol. 2012;19:4217–22.

7. Hay ID. Selective use of radioactive iodine in the postoperative management of patients with papillary and follicular thyroid carcinoma. J Surg Oncol. 2006;94:692–700.

8. Randolph GW, Duh QY, Heller KS, et al. The prognostic significance of nodal metastases from papillary thyroid carcinoma can be stratified based on the size and number of metastatic lymph nodes, as well as the presence of extranodal extension. Thyroid. 2012;22:1144–52.

9. Carling T, Carty SE, Ciarleglio MM, et al. American Thyroid Association design and feasibility of a prospective randomized controlled trial of prophylactic central lymph node dissection for papillary thyroid carcinoma. Thyroid. 2012;22:237–44.

10. Joo JY, Park JY, Yoon YH, et al. Prediction of occult central lymph node metastasis in papillary thyroid carcinoma by preoperative BRAF analysis using fine-needle aspiration biopsy: a prospective study. J Clin Endocrinol Metab. 2012;97:3996–4003.

11. Kloos RT, Eng C, Evans DB, et al. Medullary thyroid cancer: management guidelines of the American Thyroid Association. Thyroid. 2009;19:565–612.

References

1. Noguchi S, Murakami N. The value of lymph-node dissection in patients with differentiated thyroid cancer. Surg Clin North Am. 1987;67:251–61.
2. Ozaki O, Ito K, Kobayashi K, et al. Modified neck dissection for patients with nonadvanced, differentiated carcinoma of the thyroid. World J Surg. 1988;12:825–9.
3. Noguchi M, Kumaki T, Taniya T, et al. Impact of neck dissection on survival in well-differentiated thyroid cancer: a multivariate analysis of 218 cases. Int Surg. 1990;75:220–4.

4. Attie JN, Khafif RA, Steckler RM. Elective neck dissection in papillary carcinoma of the thyroid. Am J Surg. 1971;122:464–71.
5. Frankenthaler RA, Sellin RV, Cangir A, et al. Lymph node metastasis from papillary-follicular thyroid carcinoma in young patients. Am J Surg. 1990;160:341–3.
6. White ML, Gauger PG, Doherty GM. Central lymph node dissection in differentiated thyroid cancer. World J Surg. 2007;31:895–904.
7. Mulla MG, Knoefel WT, Gilbert J, et al. Lateral cervical lymph node metastases in papillary thyroid cancer: a systematic review of imaging-guided and prophylactic removal of the lateral compartment. Clin Endocrinol (Oxf). 2012;77:126–31.
8. Mazzaferri EL, Young RL, Oertel JE, et al. Papillary thyroid carcinoma: the impact of therapy in 576 patients. Medicine (Baltimore). 1977;56:171–95.
9. Coburn MC, Wanebo HJ. Prognostic factors and management considerations in patients with cervical metastases of thyroid cancer. Am J Surg. 1992;164:671–6.
10. Hamming JF, van de Velde CJ, Fleuren GJ, et al. Differentiated thyroid cancer: a stage adapted approach to the treatment of regional lymph node metastases. Eur J Cancer Clin Oncol. 1988;24:325–30.
11. Cady B, Rossi R. An expanded view of risk-group definition in differentiated thyroid carcinoma. Surgery. 1988;104:947–53.
12. Hutter RV, Frazell EL, Foote Jr FW. Elective radical neck dissection: an assessment of its use in the management of papillary thyroid cancer. CA Cancer J Clin. 1970;20:87–93.
13. McHenry CR, Rosen IB, Walfish PG. Prospective management of nodal metastases in differentiated thyroid cancer. Am J Surg. 1991;162:353–6.
14. Block MA. Management of carcinoma of the thyroid. Ann Surg. 1977;185:133–44.
15. Shah MD, Hall FT, Eski SJ, et al. Clinical course of thyroid carcinoma after neck dissection. Laryngoscope. 2003;113:2102–7.
16. Gemsenjäger E, Perren A, Seifert B, et al. Lymph node surgery in papillary thyroid carcinoma. J Am Coll Surg. 2003;197:182–90.
17. Wada N, Duh QY, Sugino K, et al. Lymph node metastasis from 259 papillary thyroid microcarcinomas. Frequency, pattern of occurrence and recurrence, and optimal strategy for neck dissection. Ann Surg. 2003;237:399–407.
18. Hillel AD, Kroll H, Dorman J, et al. Radical neck dissection: a subjective and objective evaluation of postoperative disability. J Otolaryngol. 1989;18:53–61.
19. Marchetta FC, Sako K, Matsuura H. Modified neck dissection for carcinoma of the thyroid gland. Am J Surg. 1970;120:452–5.
20. Crile Jr G. Survival of patients with papillary carcinoma of the thyroid after conservative operations. Am J Surg. 1964;108:862–6.
21. Cady B, Sedgwick CE, Meissner WA, et al. Changing clinical, pathologic, therapeutic, and survival patterns in differentiated thyroid carcinoma. Ann Surg. 1976;184:541–53.
22. Sanders LE, Rossi RL. Occult well differentiated thyroid carcinoma presenting as cervical node disease. World J Surg. 1995;19:642–6; discussion 646–7.
23. Crile Jr G. Treatment of papillary carcinoma of the thyroid with lateral cervical metastases. Am J Surg. 1950;80:419–23.
24. Mazzaferri EL, Young RL. Papillary thyroid carcinoma: a 10-year follow-up report of the impact of therapy in 576 patients. Am J Med. 1981;70:511–8.
25. McGregor GI, Luoma A, Jackson SM. Lymph node metastases from well-differentiated thyroid cancer. Am J Surg. 1985;149:610–2.
26. Musacchio MJ, Kim AW, Vijungco JD, et al. Greater local recurrence occurs with 'berry picking' than neck dissection in thyroid cancer. Am J Surg. 2003;69:191–6; discussion 196–7.
27. Palazzo F, Gosnell J, Savio R, et al. Lymphadenectomy for papillary thyroid cancer: changes in practice over four decades. Eur J Surg Oncol. 2006;32:340–4.
28. Bhattacharyya N. Surgical treatment of cervical node metastases in patients with papillary thyroid cancer. Arch Otolaryngol Head Neck Surg. 2003;129:1101–4.
29. Turanli S. Is the type of dissection in lateral neck metastases for differentiated thyroid cancer important? Otolaryngol Head Neck Surg. 2007;136:957–60.

30. Grant CS, Stulak JM, Thompson B, et al. Risks and adequacy of an optimized surgical approach to the primary surgical management of papillary thyroid carcinoma treated during 1999–2006. World J Surg. 2010;34:1239–46.
31. Farrag T, Lin F, Brownlee N, et al. Is routine dissection of level IIb and Va necessary in patients with papillary thyroid cancer undergoing lateral neck dissection for FNA-confirmed metastases in other levels? World J Surg. 2009;33:1680–3.
32. Lim YC, Choi EC, Yoon YH. Occult lymph nodes in neck level V in papillary thyroid carcinoma. Surgery. 2010;147:241–5.
33. Ahmadi N, Grewal A, Davidson B. Patterns of cervical lymph node metastases in primary and recurrent papillary thyroid cancer. J Oncol. 2011;2011:735678.
34. Caron NR, Tan YY, Ogilvie JB, et al. Selective modified radical neck dissection for papillary thyroid cancer—is level I, II and V dissection always necessary? World J Surg. 2006;30:833–40.
35. Stack Jr BC, Ferris RL, Goldenberg D. American Thyroid Association consensus review and statement regarding the anatomy, terminology, and rationale for lateral neck dissection in differentiated thyroid cancer. Thyroid. 2012;22:501–8.
36. Nason RW, Abdulrauf BM, Stranc MF. The anatomy of the accessory nerve and cervical lymph node biopsy. Am J Surg. 2000;180:241–3.
37. Sivanandan R, Soo KC. Pattern of cervical lymph node metastases from papillary carcinoma of the thyroid. Br J Surg. 2001;88:1241–4.
38. Pingpank Jr JF, Sasson AR, Hanlon AL, et al. Tumor above the spinal accessory nerve in papillary thyroid cancer that involves lateral neck nodes. Arch Otolaryngol Head Neck Surg. 2002;128:1275–8.
39. Yanir Y, Doweck I. Regional metastases in well-differentiated thyroid carcinoma: pattern of spread. Laryngoscope. 2008;118:433–6.
40. Kupferman ME, Weinstock YE, Santillan AA. Predictors of level V metastases in well differentiated thyroid cancer. Head Neck. 2008;30:1469–74.
41. Yüce I, Cağli S, Bayram A. Regional metastatic pattern of papillary thyroid carcinoma. Eur Arch Otorhinolaryngol. 2010;267:437–41.

The Management of Recurrent/ Persistent Well-Differentiated Thyroid Cancer in the Central Compartment

J.D. Pasternak and L.E. Rotstein

Introduction

The past decade has seen a marked increase within Canada in the incidence of well-differentiated thyroid cancer (WDTC). The incidence has increased 6.8 % per year in men since 1998 and 6.9 % per year in women since 2002 [1]. Once treated for WDTC, ≤20 % of patients are found to have evidence of recurrent disease [2, 3]. This recurrent disease can be seen within the central neck or elsewhere, in the lateral neck and distant sites. This chapter focuses on examining the current practice for detecting, preventing and treating recurrent WDTC in the central compartment of the neck. An overview is provided of both managing the central neck for an initial thyroid cancer operation as well as how the surgeon might diagnose and treat recurrence within it.

For the purposes of this chapter, and as is accepted widely among the surgical community, borders of the central neck are defined laterally as the carotid sheaths, superiorly as the hyoid bone, and inferiorly as the sternal notch. However, many thyroid surgeons use the brachiocephalic vessels as the inferior border. Formal central neck lymph node dissection (CNLND) for WDTC is classically described as a bilateral procedure encompassing the prelaryngeal (delphian), pretracheal and paratracheal nodal basins. A unilateral dissection, in the absence of thyroiditis, typically contains ~5–8 lymph nodes and bilateral operations have 7–17 nodes within the specimen [4].

J.D. Pasternak • L.E. Rotstein (✉)
Division of General Surgery, Toronto General Hospital, University Health Network,
200 Elizabeth Street, Toronto, ON M2G 2C4, Canada
e-mail: Lorne.Rotstein@uhn.ca

© K. Alok Pathak, Richard W. Nason, Janice L. Pasieka, Rehan Kazi,
Raghav C. Dwivedi 2015
Springer India/Byword Books
K.A. Pathak et al. (eds.), *Management of Thyroid Cancer: Special Considerations*,
Head and Neck Cancer Clinics, DOI 10.1007/978-81-322-2434-1_5

Surgery for Papillary Thyroid Cancer and Central Neck Dissection

Initial surgical management for WDTC is a topic that continues to be debated in the literature. A particularly disputed issue involves the management of the central neck at the time of thyroidectomy for WDTC in the absence of clinical evidence of level VI lymph node metastasis. Patients with diagnosed WDTC and no imaged evidence of lymph node metastasis have ≤35 % incidence of occult lymph node micrometastasis found at prophylactic CNLND [5–7]. Although ultrasound imaging is most commonly used for preoperative staging at the time of WDTC diagnosis, it not only has a notoriously low sensitivity (30–60 %) of detecting metastatic lymph node disease, but between 29 and 39 % of treated patients are upstaged because of microscopic disease found in the central neck at the time of prophylactic CNLND [5, 8–12]. This substantial risk of missing disease within the central neck at the time of curative thyroidectomy for WDTC has led to support for completing a prophylactic central neck lymph node dissection in patients with no clinical evidence of metastatic disease. The American Thyroid Association (ATA) 2006 guidelines advocated for routine central compartment lymph node dissection in all patients with papillary thyroid carcinoma [13]. This 2006 guideline has led to a debate in the literature about the specific benefits of undertaking CNLND in the absence of clinical disease versus the potential risks associated with this operation [14, 15]. That lymph node metastasis of WDTC does not specifically affect survival and might have a minimal affect on recurrence, especially when considering prognostic scoring systems for WDTC, has been backed by good evidence [16–20]. On the other hand, inherent risks of central neck dissection even on 'untouched tissues' include those to the voice and calcium homeostasis.

Risks

As previously mentioned, the two main risks of a bilateral prophylactic CNLND include hypoparathyroidism and recurrent laryngeal nerve (RLN) injury. Hypoparathyroidism may result from the devascularization of the parathyroid glands, which are usually confined to the borders of the central compartment. Even with adequate autotransplantation, transient hypocalcaemia may be clinically severe and unsuccessful autotransplantation is a risk. Opinions differ on what the true incidence of hypoparathyroidism is after prophylactic CNLND, but many surgeons agree that a bilateral CNLND is associated with higher rates of transient hypoparathyroidism [21]. The evidence for risk of damage to the RLN is less clear. Palestini et al. showed that patients who had prophylactic bilateral neck dissection had a higher rate of transient RLN paralysis when compared to patients who had a total thyroidectomy alone (7.8 vs. 1.3) [22]. As a result, the ATA revised its guidelines in 2009, changing its position on prophylactic CNLND. These guidelines now support that central neck dissection should be performed in patients with clinically evident nodal metastasis and may be prophylactically considered for more advanced primary tumours (T3 and T4) in the setting of no preoperative evidence of positive nodes [3]. Due to current literaire showing small increases in morbidity for bilateral CNLND and the low risk (9 %) of a skip metastasis to the contralateral central neck, there has been an increase in advocacy for only prophylactic unilateral CNLND when appropriate [23].

Detecting Recurrent Papillary Thyroid Cancer and the Central Neck

The ATA guidelines suggest that patients should be followed after thyroid cancer with clinical examination, imaging (ultrasound is most often used) and serial serum thyroglobulin (Tg). It is difficult to determine if detectable recurrent disease, especially within the first few months after initial operative intervention is, in fact, persistent. Newer understanding of aggressive recurrent tumour biology and better detection of persistent disease helps the surgeon determine prognosis [24]. Regardless, clinically or radiologically detectable disease within the central neck is an indication for therapeutic CNLND even after previous thyroid surgery. The ATA guidelines have explained that the risk to the parathyroid glands and RLN would be justified with imaged or palpable disease [3]. Notably, Alvarado et al. have published on a sample of patients who underwent completion thyroidectomy after diagnostic hemithyroidectomy for subsequently confirmed WDTC [25]. They performed a prophylactic central neck dissection at the time of completion hemithyroidectomy, noting ≥60 % prevalence of lymph node metastasis with a negligible increased risk to the RLN and parathyroids [25].

Imaging

Currently, most surgeons use neck ultrasonography as the imaging modality of choice for screening detection of recurrent disease in the central neck [3]. Once nodal disease is discovered, further imaging is often used for preoperative planning and to ensure that all disease is identified for curative resection. Alternative imaging options include computed tomography (CT) with and without iodinated contrast, magnetic resonance imaging (MRI) and positron emission tomography (PET). CT with contrast is considered to be sensitive for delineating the anatomy preoperatively as well as confirming the presence of central lymph node metastasis [26]. Some authors avoid contrast because of concerns regarding iodine stunning delaying potential therapeutic radioiodine administration. Qiu et al. have reported using I^{131} contrast SPECT-CT to detect parapharyngeal metastasis, which could help in localizing iodine-sensitive thyroid cancer metastasis [27]. Growing opinion suggests that PET scans are not as helpful as initially thought, in that they do not add much localization benefit [26]. Other less helpful imaging modalities include MRI, which is thought to be less useful in characterizing central neck recurrence caused by oesophageal movement artifact. Intraoperative radioactive iodine detection has been used in a study of 31 patients to localize disease with a gamma probe [28]. Charcoal tattoo and other systems, such as intraoperative ultrasound-guided methylene blue dye localization systems, have been shown to provide good localization as well [29, 30]. Surgeon-performed ultrasound and intraoperative technetium tracing have been used with good results to localize nodal disease before reoperation [31]. Currently, most endocrine surgeons employ the use of ultrasonography initially for detection of recurrent disease within the central neck; however, when additional imaging is employed, CT has been shown to be more robust than MRI in detecting metastatic deposits in the neck [3, 32].

Biochemical Detection

A lack of consensus remains on the type of tumour marker to follow and its optimal level after surgery for WDTC. Many thyroidologists aim for the most sensitive marker of cure, specifically a thyroid stimulating hormone (TSH)-stimulated undetectable Tg level while others, on the other hand, tolerate low circulating basal Tg levels without attempting to intervene [33]. The debate of how to follow Tg levels and when they should be TSH-stimulated is beyond the focus of this chapter. Reoperation within the central neck, however, is reserved for when persistent or recurrent disease is clinically or radiologically evident, and/or with some biochemical evidence of disease persistence/progression. Interestingly, biochemical evidence is not mandatory for reoperation, as apparent in Clayman's group of reoperative central neck dissections [34]. Twenty-six per cent of patients with pathologically confirmed metastasis had a Tg level of <3. Moreover, currently no recommendations have been made for central neck exploration without good imaging evidence of disease in patients with high tumour markers. A caveat to this idea is that lymph nodes in the central neck might meet lesser imaging diagnostic criteria than elsewhere in and outside the neck, given a positive tumour marker. More varied forms of axial imaging, such as CT, may be used to investigate recurrence, even in the presence of low Tg levels. CT criteria of suspicious lymph nodal metastasis include dense cortical enhancement that is more than that of adjacent muscles, calcifications, size or cystic or necrotic change [35].

Treatment Options for Central Compartment Recurrence

Operative intervention for recurrent nodal disease of WDTC in the central neck is by definition a reoperation, assuming the patient was treated with a form of thyroidectomy for the primary tumour. Whereas this operation is usually done with curative intent, situations arise in which a palliative dissection is carried out. In the case of airway compression and distant metastasis, a CNLND may be performed to decrease the burden of disease. Mostly, however, resection of evident central lymph nodes is performed with a therapeutic reoperative, oncological goal. Regardless of intent, any second operation in the neck carries with it increased risks when compared to

Table 5.1 Complications after reoperative central compartment (level VI) lymph node dissection

Author/Year	Study information	RLN palsy		Hypocalcaemia	
		Transient (%)	Permanent (%)	Transient (%)	Permanent (%)
Shah et al. (2012) [42]	82 pts retrospective review	2	2	20	7
Clayman et al. (2009) [34]	63 pts retrospective review	2	0	19	18[b]
Alvarado et al. (2009) [25]	193 pts retrospective review	3	0.6	11	2
Farrag et al. (2006) [47]	33 pts retrospective review	21	0	6	0
Tufano et al. (2012) [45]	120 pts retrospective review		14.2[a]	10	2.5
Shen et al. (2010) [48]	106 pts retrospective review	4.7	1.9	23.6	0.9
Lang et al. (2013) [49]	50 pts retrospective review	6	1	14	0

[a]RLN resected due to tumour burden
[b]Permanent + persistent
RLN recurrent laryngeal nerve, *pts* patients

operating on any untouched tissues. The central neck has its own set of unique anatomical challenges with reoperation.

Assuming the parathyroid glands have been left *in situ* and the RLNs were not damaged from the initial thyroid cancer treatment, scar and distorted anatomy have been seen to increase risks of injury to these structures compared to surgery on necks which have never had an operation [36]. As previously noted, the risks to these structures that are inherent to CNLND are amplified by reoperation. Table 5.1 shows reported hypoparathyroidism and RLN palsy postoperatively for CNLND. Most studies report a modest rate of transient RLN palsy. However, transient hypocalcaemia rates of between 6 % and 23.6 % can lead to substantial morbidity for patients (Table 5.1). As Steward describes in his review of thyroid cancer reoperation, a publication bias might exist wherein only the best thyroid surgeons are reporting their complication rates, implying that there may be groups of patients who are facing much higher complication rates from central neck reoperations [6].

As an interesting alternative to surgery for detected central neck recurrence of WDTC, some centres select patients with low recurrent tumour burden for percutaneous ethanol injection into metastatic lymph nodes. Whereas this method might decrease the risks of reoperation, debate still exists if it is oncologically sound. Also, there are concerns regarding fibrosis generation precluding potential reoperation, if this is required subsequently. Heilo et al. report treating 109 patients with percutaneous ethanol injection and having a 93 % response rate with 66 % of nodes disappearing after a mean follow up of 3 years [37]. Kim et al. reported a similar series with 27 patients [38]. Nevertheless, given its potential clinical value, the efficacy of this therapy needs more validation before it can be widely adopted [39].

Operative Conduct

It was relatively recently that thyroid surgeons believed reoperation in the central neck was acceptable, given the risks [40]. It is imperative that before any reoperation, the function of the RLNs as well as location of the remaining parathyroid glands be confirmed and documented. Incision for reoperative is usually positioned on the previous thyroidectomy scar in the lower neck. The incision may have to be extended laterally on the side of disease for easier visualization. When re-elevating the subplatysmal flaps and freeing the strap muscles in the midline substantial fibrosis is often revealed, especially if haemostatic agents were previously employed. The RLN and parathyroid pedical identification and preservation are crucial to a central neck reoperative setting. Evidence shows that RLN monitoring may help the surgeon distinguish fibrotic areas close to the nerve from recurrent disease [41]. Some surgeons identify the RLN from a previously undissected region vis-a-vis the lateral or lower neck [36]. The personal preference of the present authors is to define the common carotid artery from the thoracic outlet to the level of the cricoid and then attempt to identify the RLN as low as possible in the paratracheal position in the superior mediastinum. The RLN must be followed from its entry into the operative field towards its cephalic location, staying on the anteromedial border of it. An alternative to continuous nerve monitoring is to use intermittent nerve stimulation to confirm function in the absence of long-acting muscle relaxants. Visualizing the remaining inferior thyroid artery may help to identify the main pedicles to the parathyroid glands. The inferior gland is likely to be sacrificed as a result of scar/tumour involvement. The superior parathyroid is usually above the RLN angle and not at as much risk. Any devascularized (dark brown/black) parathyroid gland is excised and preserved for autotransplantation after histological confirmation. Once the surgeon is confident of the identification and preservation of these structures, resection of all lymph nodes within the borders of the central neck may ensue. Identifying the surfaces of the trachea also helps with identifying existing disease. A comprehensive resection is performed on the ipsilateral side, removing all nodal tissue in the area from the trachea to the carotid and from the cricoid down to the innominate artery. Attention must be paid to ensure that all macroscopic disease in level VII is detected and excised as well. A decision with respect to contralateral dissection is made at this juncture. Some authors recommend bilateral excision at the time of this procedure; others, including the present authors, will only perform bilateral central dissections if documented evidence exists of contralateral disease and the RLN on the first side has been identified and deemed functional. If lateral masses or lymph nodes are palpable, a more extensive operation is considered.

Outcomes

Reoperating in the central neck for recurrent WDTC has varied reported outcomes. Clayman et al. report that 71 % of patients had their Tg reduced to undetectable levels [34]. Shah et al. report normalization (≤ 2 ng/ml) of Tg in only 56 % of patients [42]. Both studies followed patients for 18 and 28 months, respectively. Other studies looking at both the central neck as well as reoperation in the lateral neck show similar response rates to those mentioned above [43, 44]. Aggressiveness of disease as predicted by time to recurrence, burden and subtype of tumour and level and trajectory of Tg marker determine outcomes for re-recurrence of disease.

Future Directions

CNLND and treatment of recurrence continue to cause much debate among thyroidologists. With improved detection of occult disease and further biochemical analysis of thyroid tumours, the surgeon may better predict response to intervention. Tufano et al. correlated BRAF genetic mutated tumour status with the length of time to central neck recurrence from the initial operation [45]. Those individuals with the mutation had a shorter time to reoperation and a higher number of metastatic central neck lymph nodes [46]. With further knowledge of this disease at a molecular and genetic level, we can begin to stratify patients with worse tumour prognosis to more aggressive surgical management. Disease-free survival is an appropriate marker to use when evaluating the effectiveness of surgical intervention. The obstacle, however, is in following patients long enough to account for the indolent nature of WDTC.

Commentary

Richard W. Nason

The fact that well-differentiated thyroid cancer (WDTC) is relatively rare and has a protected course with a relatively low mortality rate means that there can be a great variability in treatment without any appreciable change in mortality. There is, therefore, controversy in the management of many aspects of this cancer, and this includes the timing and extent of surgery for cervical lymph node metastases in the central compartment. Badly treated thyroid cancer leads to recurrence and disease progression with significant morbidity and potential mortality. The initial surgical management is critical to the success in management of this disease. In the absence of controlled trials to guide treatment, management is based on what is known about the natural history of the disease as garnered from clinical experience.

The initial site of lymph node metastases in WDTC is the central compartment and involvement of lymph nodes is common. The significance of occult metastases, in the authors' opinion, is unresolved. The problem in the elective management of the central compartment lies in balancing the risk of recurrence against the risks of surgical treatment. These issues are prominent in both the timing and extent of surgical dissection. The timing of elective neck dissection is addressed by the American Thyroid Association (ATA) guidelines. As described in this chapter, the ATA guidelines of 2006 advocated routine central compartment lymph node dissection in patients with WDTC. More recent, revised ATA guidelines (2009) state that prophylactic central compartment neck dissection may be performed in patients with papillary thyroid carcinoma with clinically uninvolved central neck lymph nodes, especially for advanced primary tumours (T3 or T4). The more recent position reflects the lack of evidence for improved outcome with elective central compartment node dissection and recognition of increased complications when the procedure is performed. With respect to the extent of elective treatment, evidence supports the relatively infrequent incidence of contralateral metastases in the absence of gross lymph node involvement.

The above considerations have influenced the authors' approach to the central compartment in WDTC. It is important to emphasize that clinical assessment and current imaging modalities are inaccurate in determining the status of the central compartment lymph nodes. The best way to assess these lymph nodes is at the time of surgery with the central compartment exposed. Involved lymph nodes are addressed with a compartment-orientated dissection, as detailed elsewhere in this monograph. Ipsilateral elective dissection is considered with advanced primary tumours.

If it is elected to observe the central compartment, then reoperation in this area will be inevitable in a small percentage of patients. The key to successful management of recurrence in the central compartment includes a thorough understanding of the anatomy of the recurrent laryngeal nerve and its variations, a lateral and low approach to identifying the recurrent laryngeal nerve, and the surgeon's experience.

References

1. Canadian Cancer Society's Steering Committee on Cancer Statistics. Canadian cancer statistics 2012. Toronto: Canadian Cancer Society; 2012.
2. Enewold L, Zhu K, Ron E, et al. Rising thyroid cancer incidence in the United States by demographic and tumor characteristics, 1980–2005. Cancer Epidemiol Biomarkers Prev. 2009;18:784–91.
3. American Thyroid Association (ATA) Guidelines Taskforce on Thyroid Nodules and Differentiated Thyroid Cancer, Cooper DS, Doherty GM, Haugen BR, et al. Revised American Thyroid Association management guidelines for patients with thyroid nodules and differentiated thyroid cancer. Thyroid. 2009;19:1167–214.
4. Hartl DM, Leboulleux S, Al Ghuzlan A, et al. Optimization of staging of the neck with prophylactic central and lateral neck dissection for papillary thyroid carcinoma. Ann Surg. 2012;255:777–83.
5. Randolph G, Duh QY, Heller KS, et al. The prognostic significance of nodal metastases from papillary thyroid carcinoma can be stratified based on the size and number of metastatic lymph nodes, as well as the presence of extranodal extension: ATA Surgical Affairs Committee's Taskforce on Thyroid Cancer Nodal Surgery. Thyroid. 2012;10.
6. Steward DL. Update in utility of secondary node dissection for papillary thyroid cancer. J Clin Endocrinol Metab. 2012;97:3393–8.

7. Lee KE, Chung IY, Kang E, et al. Ipsilateral and contralateral central lymph node metastasis in papillary thyroid cancer: Patterns and predictive factors of nodal metastasis. Head Neck. 2013;35:672–6.
8. Mulla M, Schulte KM. Central cervical lymph node metastases in papillary thyroid cancer: a systematic review of imaging-guided and prophylactic removal of the central compartment. Clin Endocrinol (Oxf). 2012;76:131–6.
9. Sywak M, Cornford L, Roach P, et al. Routine ipsilateral level VI lymphadenectomy reduces postoperative thyroglobulin levels in papillary thyroid cancer. Surgery. 2006;140:1000–100.
10. Choi JS, Kim J, Kwak JY, et al. Preoperative staging of papillary thyroid carcinoma: comparison of ultrasound imaging and CT. AJR Am J Roentgenol. 2009;193:871–8.
11. Hughes DT, White ML, Miller BS, et al. Influence of prophylactic central lymph node dissection on postoperative thyroglobulin levels and radioiodine treatment in papillary thyroid cancer. Surgery. 2010;148:1100–6; discussion 1006–7.
12. Shindo M, Wu JC, Park EE, et al. The importance of central compartment elective lymph node excision in the staging and treatment of papillary thyroid cancer. Arch Otolaryngol Head Neck Surg. 2006;132:650–4.
13. Cooper DS, Doherty GM, Haugen BR, et al. The American Thyroid Association Guidelines Taskforce. Management guidelines for patients with thyroid nodules and differentiated thyroid cancer. Thyroid. 2006;16:109–42.
14. Cheah WK, Arici C, Ituarte PH, et al. Complications of neck dissection for thyroid cancer. World J Surg. 2002;26:1013–6.
15. White ML, Gauger PG, Doherty GM. Central lymph node dissection in differentiated thyroid cancer. World J Surg. 2007;31:895–904.
16. Hay ID, Bergstralh EJ, Goellner JR, et al. Predicting outcome in papillary thyroid carcinoma: development of a reliable prognostic scoring system in a cohort of 1779 patients surgically treated at one institution during 1940 through 1989. Surgery. 1993;114:1050–8.
17. Cady B, Rossi R. An expanded view of risk-group definition in differentiated thyroid carcinoma. Surgery. 1988;104:947–53.
18. DeGroot LJ, Kaplan EL, McCormick M, et al. Natural history, treatment, and course of papillary thyroid carcinoma. J Clin Endocrinol Metab. 1990;71:414–24.
19. Mazzaferri EL, Jhiang SM. Long-term impact of initial surgical and medical therapy on papillary and follicular thyroid cancer. Am J Med. 1994;97:418–28.
20. Shaha AR, Loree TR, Shah JP. Intermediate-risk group for differentiated carcinoma of the thyroid. Surgery. 1994;116:1036–41.
21. Giordano D, Valcavi R, Thompson GB, et al. Complications of central neck dissection in patients with papillary thyroid carcinoma: Results of a study on 1087 patients and review of the literature. Thyroid. 2012;22:911–7.
22. Palestini N, Borasi A, Cestino L, et al. Is central neck dissection a safe procedure in the treatment of papillary thyroid cancer? Our experience. Langenbecks Arch Surg. 2008;393:693–8.
23. Lim YC, Koo BS. Predictive factors of skip metastases to lateral neck compartment leaping central neck compartment in papillary thyroid carcinoma. Oral Oncol. 2012;48:262–5.
24. Lin JD, Hsueh C, Chao TC. Early recurrence of papillary and follicular thyroid carcinoma predicts a worse outcome. Thyroid. 2009;19:1053–9.
25. Alvarado R, Sywak MS, Delbridge L, et al. Central lymph node dissection as a secondary procedure for papillary thyroid cancer: Is there added morbidity? Surgery. 2009;145:514–8.
26. Choi JW, Lee JH, Baek JH, et al. Diagnostic accuracy of ultrasound and 18-F-FDG PET or PET/CT for patients with suspected recurrent papillary thyroid carcinoma. Ultrasound Med Biol. 2010;36:1608–15.
27. Qiu ZL, Xu YH, Song HJ, et al. Localization and identification of parapharyngeal metastases from differentiated thyroid carcinoma by 131I-SPECT/CT. Head Neck. 2011;33:171–7.
28. Rubello D, Salvatori M, Ardito G, et al. Iodine-131 radio-guided surgery in differentiated thyroid cancer: Outcome on 31 patients and review of the literature. Biomed Pharmacother. 2007;61:477–81.

29. Soprani F, Bondi F, Puccetti M, et al. Charcoal tattoo localization for differentiated thyroid cancer recurrence in the central compartment of the neck. Acta Otorhinolaryngol Ital. 2012;32:87–92.

30. Harari A, Sippel RS, Goldstein R, et al. Successful localization of recurrent thyroid cancer in reoperative neck surgery using ultrasound-guided methylene blue dye injection. J Am Coll Surg. 2012;215:555–61.

31. Erbil Y, Sari S, Adcaodlu O, et al. Radio-guided excision of metastatic lymph nodes in thyroid carcinoma: a safe technique for previously operated neck compartments. World J Surg. 2010;34:2581–8.

32. Schuff KG, Weber SM, Givi B, et al. Efficacy of nodal dissection for treatment of persistent/ recurrent papillary thyroid cancer. Laryngoscope. 2008;118:768–75.

33. Benbassat CA, Mechlis-Frish S, Guttmann H, et al. Current concepts in the follow-up of patients with differentiated thyroid cancer. Isr Med Assoc J. 2007;9:540–5.

34. Clayman GL, Shellenberger TD, Ginsberg LE, et al. Approach and safety of comprehensive central compartment dissection in patients with recurrent papillary thyroid carcinoma. Head Neck. 2009;31:1152–63.

35. Yoon JH, Kim JY, Moon HJ, et al. Contribution of computed tomography to ultrasound in predicting lateral lymph node metastasis in patients with papillary thyroid carcinoma. Ann Surg Oncol. 2011;18:1734–41.

36. Moley JF, Lairmore TC, Doherty GM, et al. Preservation of the recurrent laryngeal nerves in thyroid and parathyroid reoperations. Surgery. 1999;126:673–7; discussion 677–9.

37. Heilo A, Sigstad E, Fagerlid KH, et al. Efficacy of ultrasound-guided percutaneous ethanol injection treatment in patients with a limited number of metastatic cervical lymph nodes from papillary thyroid carcinoma. J Clin Endocrinol Metab. 2011;96:2750–5.

38. Kim BM, Kim MJ, Kim EK, et al. Controlling recurrent papillary thyroid carcinoma in the neck by ultrasonography-guided percutaneous ethanol injection. Eur Radiol. 2008;18:835–42.

39. Lewis BD, Hay ID, Charboneau JW, et al. Percutaneous ethanol injection for treatment of cervical lymph node metastases in patients with papillary thyroid carcinoma. AJR Am J Roentgenol. 2002;178:699–704.

40. Levin KE, Clark AH, Duh QY, et al. Reoperative thyroid surgery. Surgery. 1992;111:604–9.

41. Kim MK, Mandel SH, Baloch Z, et al. Morbidity following central compartment reoperation for recurrent or persistent thyroid cancer. Arch Otolaryngol Head Neck Surg. 2004;130:1214–6.

42. Shah MD, Harris LD, Nassif RG, et al. Efficacy and safety of central compartment neck dissection for recurrent thyroid carcinoma. Arch Otolaryngol Head Neck Surg. 2012;138:33–7.

43. Roh JL, Kim JM, Park CI. Central compartment reoperation for recurrent/persistent differentiated thyroid cancer: patterns of recurrence, morbidity, and prediction of postoperative hypocalcemia. Ann Surg Oncol. 2011;18:1312–8.

44. Pai SI, Tufano RP. Reoperation for recurrent/persistent well-differentiated thyroid cancer. Otolaryngol Clin North Am. 2010;43:353–63.

45. Tufano RP, Bishop J, Wu G. Reoperative central compartment dissection for patients with recurrent/persistent papillary thyroid cancer: efficacy, safety, and the association of the BRAF mutation. Laryngoscope. 2012;122:1634–40.

46. Hughes DT, Laird AM, Miller BS, et al. Reoperative lymph node dissection for recurrent papillary thyroid cancer and effect on serum thyroglobulin. Ann Surg Oncol. 2012;19:2951–7.

47. Farrag TY, Agrawal N, Sheth S, et al. Algorithm for safe and effective reoperative thyroid bed surgery for recurrent/persistent papillary thyroid carcinoma. Head Neck. 2007;29:1069–74.

48. Shen WT, Ogawa L, Ruan D, et al. Central neck lymph node dissection for papillary thyroid cancer: comparison of complication and recurrence rates in 295 initial dissections and reoperations. Arch Surg. 2010;145:272–5.

49. Lang BH, Lee GC, Ng CP, et al. Evaluating the morbidity and efficacy of reoperative surgery in the central compartment for persistent/recurrent papillary thyroid carcinoma. World J Surg. 2013;37:2853–9.

Management of Distant Metastases in Differentiated Thyroid Cancer

Adrian Harvey

Introduction

Follicular cell-derived differentiated thyroid cancer (DTC) is a disease character-ized by long-term survival and excellent prognosis. Large-scale studies have defined 10-year survival rates of 85 % in follicular thyroid cancer (FTC) and ~93 % in papil-lary thyroid cancer (PTC) [1–5]. Despite this, published series report that 6–20 % of patients will develop distant metastatic disease [3, 4, 6–16]. Outcomes in these patients with distant disease are significantly worse, with 10-year survival rates closely approximating 40 % [3, 4, 6, 7, 9, 10, 12–23]. Numerous risk factors have been linked to the development of both regional and distant disease. These include age, tumour size, extrathyroidal extension, multifocality and palpable lymphade-nopathy [3, 8, 11, 24]. In 5–45 % of patients, distant disease will be discovered at the time of initial diagnosis on cross-sectional imaging or post-therapy radioactive iodine (RAI) scans [1, 6, 15, 18, 19, 22, 25, 26]. The remainder of patients will develop metastatic recurrence during follow-up. In this latter group, distant disease may be discovered more than 10 years after the initial treatment.

Distant metastases occur outside the thyroid bed and regional lymph node basins. The most common sites in DTC are the lung and bone [6, 7, 9–13, 18, 22]. A small number of patients will also develop metastases in areas other than these. Atypical sites include the brain, skin and liver, with rare reports of spread to the gastrointes-tinal tract, adrenals, uterus and omentum [6, 9, 22, 27–29]. Multiple sites of disease are found in <25 % of patients [6, 10, 12, 13, 18, 22]. This chapter discusses the prog-nosis in patients with distant metastatic disease, diagnosis and treatment options.

A. Harvey
Department of Surgery, Faculty of Medicine, University of Calgary, Calgary, AB, Canada
e-mail: Adrian.Harvey@albertahealthservices.ca

© K. Alok Pathak, Richard W. Nason, Janice L. Pasieka, Rehan Kazi,
Raghav C. Dwivedi 2015
Springer India/Byword Books
K.A. Pathak et al. (eds.), *Management of Thyroid Cancer: Special Considerations*,
Head and Neck Cancer Clinics, DOI 10.1007/978-81-322-2434-1_6

Prognosis

Prognosis in patients with distant metastatic disease is comparatively poor, with 10-year overall survival rates of ~40 %. However, this figure probably represents an overgeneralization of a highly heterogeneous group. Numerous series have defined prognostic factors that appear to significantly influence the outcome in these patients [6, 7, 9, 10, 13, 15–19, 22, 23, 30]. These indicators can be used to define subsets of patients in whom the long-term overall survival ranges from <10 to >90 %. A review of the relevant literature reveals a wide range of potential prognostic factors in metastatic DTC, most of which can be grouped into the following categories: (i) patient-, (ii) tumour-, and (iii) treatment-related variables (Table 6.1). Given the relative rarity of advanced disease in this patient population, many published reports are limited by the lack of sufficient power to perform multivariate analysis on a significant number of factors.

Patient Factors

As is the case with primary treatment of localized DTC, age has proven to be a powerful prognostic indicator in patients with more extensive disease. In a series of 336 patients with distant metastases, Shoup et al. reported that an age of <45 years was associated with a 10-year disease-specific survival of 58 % compared with just 13 % in older patients [22]. Similar findings were published by Durante et al. in 2006 on a series of 444 patients [18]. The powerful impact of age is illustrated by smaller series in which it is often one of the only prognostic variables that consistently stands up to multivariate analysis [13, 16, 31]. In contrast to age, the evidence

Table 6.1 Supporting literature for prognostic factors in metastatic differentiated thyroid cancer

Factor	Literature (references)	
	Univariate	Multivariate
Patient (references)		
Age	(17, 33)	(7, 13, 15, 16, 18, 22, 31)
Gender	NS	(18)
Tumour (references)		
Histology	(7, 17)	(15, 31)
Site	(15, 23)	(7, 13, 17, 18, 22, 31, 33, 35)
Pattern	(13)	(17, 18)
Symptoms	NS	(22)
Timing	NS	(33)
Tg	NS	NS
Treatment (references)		
RAI avidity	(13, 23)	(7, 15, 17, 18, 22, 33, 35)
RAI response	NS	(18)

NS not significant, *RAI* radioactive iodine, *Tg* thyroglobulin supporting the prognostic significance of gender is more variable. Whereas most series have failed to demonstrate significant outcome differences between men and women on multivariate analysis, Durante et al. reported a lower relative risk of death in women (RR=0.7 [0.6–0.9]; p<0.008) [18].

Tumour Factors

Numerous tumour factors have also been linked to prognosis. In particular, the site of metastatic disease appears to dictate outcome. As previously mentioned, the most common site of metastatic disease in DTC is the lung. Up to 75 % of patients will have pulmonary metastases and 40–55 % will have the lung as the only site of disease [6, 7, 15, 18, 22]. Nixon et al., in a review of 52 patients with metastatic DTC found that extrapulmonary metastases were associated with a lower overall 5–year survival (46 % vs. 75 %; p<0.13) [31]. In addition, Durante et al. found that patients with lung-only disease were more likely to achieve negative imaging after RAI treatment, a pattern associated with 10-year survival in excess of 90 % [18]. This finding is somewhat surprising, given that the most commonly reported cause of death in thyroid cancer is respiratory failure secondary to replacement of lung tissue by cancer [26, 32]. Some authors have suggested that the pattern of lung disease may influence survival [17]. Micronodular, diffuse patterns (Fig. 6.1a, b) appear to be more favourable than macronodular disease (Fig. 6.2a, b), or associated mediastinal lymphadenopathy and/or effusion. Indeed, patients with micronodular disease were more common among those who achieved negative imaging after treatment in the aforementioned series by Durante et al. [18].

Approximately 45 % of patients with metastatic DTC will have skeletal involvement [7, 13, 18, 22, 25, 33, 34]. Of these, bone is the only site in 25–40 %. The most common sites for bone metastases are the vertebrae, pelvis, ribs and femur. Published survival rates at 10 years vary from 15 to 38 % [7, 13, 18, 22, 25, 33–35]. Whereas this appears lower than survival rates published for pulmonary metastases, a number of large series have failed to establish significant differences in outcomes. In addition, bone disease is a direct cause of death in only a fraction of these patients [2, 25, 26, 32]. Therefore, it may be that bone disease simply reflects more advanced/resistant disease.

A smaller proportion of patients (12–20 %) will have multiple sites of disease [6, 18, 22]. Multiple sites of metastatic disease are not, surprisingly, associated with poor outcome. Shoup et al. reported a 17 % 10-year survival with two or more sites of metastatic disease compared with 32 % for lung-only and 27 % for bone-only metastases, a difference supported by multivariate analysis on 336 patients (p<0.0001) [22].

Primary tumour histology might also be linked to prognosis in metastatic disease. Similar to the trend seen in overall survival for primary disease, patients with metastatic disease from FTC may fare more poorly than those with papillary subtypes. Sampson et al. reported a 3-year survival of 75 % for PTC metastases

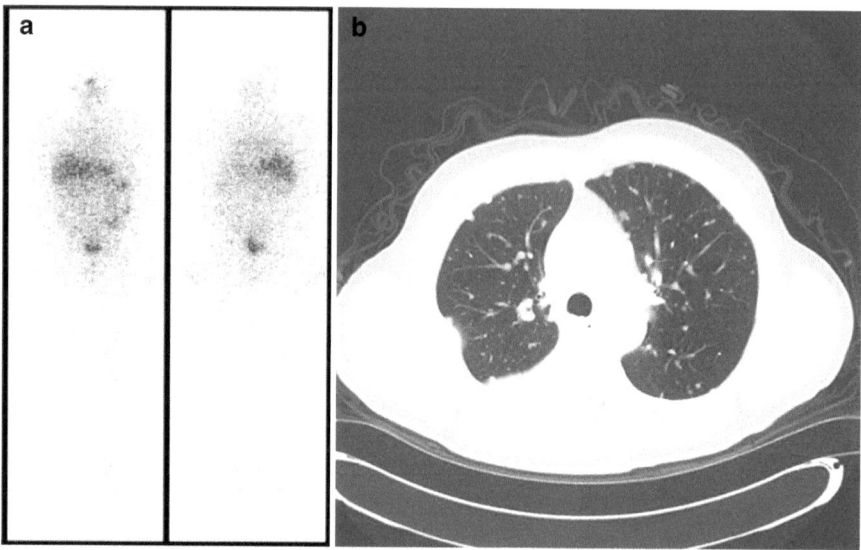

Fig. 6.1 (**a**) Radioactive iodine scan in a patient with micronodular lung disease. Increased diffuse uptake is seen throughout the lung fields. (**b**) CT scan in a patient with micronodular (<1 cm) lung metastases

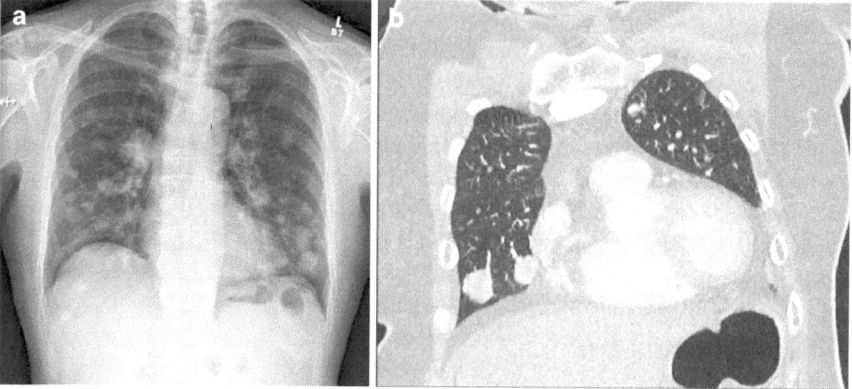

Fig. 6.2 (**a**) Chest X-ray in a patient with macronodular lung metastases. (**b**) CT scan in a patient with macronodular lung metastases

compared with 62 % for FTC (p < 0.006) [15]. However, larger series have found no such effect or findings that disappear on multivariate analysis. This observation may result from confounding factors, such as an increase in bone metastases in FTC as well as diminished avidity for and response to RAI [15, 18].

The presentation of metastatic DTC has also been examined for its potential significance. The following factors have been evaluated: (i) the timing of metastases (synchronous vs. metachronous), (ii) the presence of concomitant neck recurrence; (iii) the presence of clinical symptoms, etc. [6, 15, 16, 18, 22] None of these appear consistently to impact outcome in these patients. Finally, serum thyroglobulin (Tg) at diagnosis has been investigated, but any effect seems to disappear with multivariate analysis, suggesting this is simply a surrogate marker for other factors [15, 18].

Treatment Factors

Treatment-related factors have also proven to provide significant prognostic information. One of the most powerful variables studied appears to be the avidity of the disease for RAI and its subsequent response to therapy. Durante et al. identified three subsets of patients with respect to RAI avidity and response to treatment: (i) those with RAI-avid disease and negative imaging after treatment; (ii) RAI-avid disease but unable to achieve negative imaging with therapy; and (iii) no RAI avidity at diagnosis [18]. The 10-year survival rates for these groups were markedly different at 92 %, 29 % and 10 %, respectively [18]. Although still significant, not surprisingly, a number of confounding factors contributed to this large difference in prognosis. Specifically, patients in the most favourable group were more likely to be <40 years of age, have PTC and micronodular lung-only disease. Similarly, Casara et al. found RAI uptake to be an independent predictor of outcome in a review of 214 patients with metastatic DTC [7].

Summary

In summary, metastatic DTC has considerably worse overall outcomes compared to localized disease with survival estimated at ~40 % over 10 years. However, considerable variability exists within this group with respect to response to treatment and outcome. Young patients (<40 years) with lung-only, micronodular disease that is RAI-avid might have 10-year survival rates of >90 %. In contrast, older patients with multi-organ metastases and negative RAI scans have an expected long-term survival closer to 10 %. Clinicians involved in the care of these patients should consider these variables in advising prognosis and planning treatment strategies.

Diagnosis of Metastatic Disease

As previously noted, in 5–45 % of patients with distant disease, metastases are diagnosed at the time of initial presentation [1, 6, 15, 18, 19, 22, 25, 26]. In these patients the extent of disease becomes evident on preoperative cross-sectional imaging or post-therapeutic RAI scans. In a small percentage of patients, the metastatic disease itself is the initial presentation of DTC [9, 12, 15, 16, 19, 31, 36]. The remaining patients will have their metastatic disease discovered during routine follow-up.

Long-term follow-up in DTC is crucial, as recurrence may occur 10–20 years after initial treatment. Post-cancer surveillance recommendations rely heavily on neck ultrasound and serum Tg measurements [1]. Diagnostic RAI scans are used selectively in specific patients. The emphasis on neck imaging is supported by the observation that most recurrences are located in regional nodal basins [1, 3, 4]. However, a rising Tg with negative neck imaging suggests the possibility of distant metastatic disease.

An elevated serum Tg with no evidence of regional recurrence is appropriately investigated by diagnostic RAI scanning [1]. Unfortunately, 10–15 % of such patients will have a negative scan [1, 37–42]. This lack of sensitivity could result from insufficient dosing or problems in patient preparation with respect to thyroid hormone withdrawal or low iodine diet [37, 38]. Truly negative scans in this setting may be a consequence of tumour dedifferentiation with loss of cell membrane expression of the sodium-iodide symporter [12, 37, 38, 43–47].

Subsequent work up in these patients is somewhat controversial. Use of cross-sectional imaging and traditional radiographs in this setting is limited by poor sensitivity. Some authors have supported the routine administration of therapeutic-dose RAI [41, 42, 48]. Pacini et al. found evidence of uptake on 30/42 patients with elevated Tg and negative diagnostic scans following administration of therapeutic doses (90–150 mCi) [42]. Similarly, Pineda et al. demonstrated metastatic disease on post-therapy scans (150–300 mCi) in 16/17 patients [48]. Unfortunately, neither report could show any impact on outcomes. A recent review concluded that whereas it is not uncommon for uptake to be demonstrated with a therapeutic dose, evidence of clinical benefit is insufficient to recommend this practice [40].

Recently, the utility of FDG PET/SPECT in these patients has been examined [49–56]. Routine use of this expensive, limited resource is not justified, given the low risk of metastases and its limited sensitivity when applied broadly. Wang et al. performed both RAI and FDG SPECT in 239 patients being followed for DTC [54]. The overall sensitivities of both RAI scanning and FDG SPECT in patients with elevated Tg were just 48.7 % and 50.4 %, respectively. However, a 'flip-flop' phenomena was noted in which FDG SPECT was more likely to be positive in the setting of a negative RAI scan. In fact, the sensitivity of FDG SPECT was significantly higher in this setting (89.7 %) compared to when these traditional tests were positive (18.6 %). Similar findings have also been reported by a number of other authors [49, 57]. Schluter et al. demonstrated that the accuracy of FDG PET appears to be correlated with increasing serum Tg levels [53]. In this series, true positive rates were 11 %, 50 % and 93 % in the setting of Tg levels of <10, 10–20 and >100 ug/L, respectively. Given this, the authors suggested that this test is more appropriately targeted to those patients with a serum Tg of >10 ug/L.

The use of FDG PET/SPECT may also provide prognostic information and guide treatment. Unfortunately, non-iodine avid, FDG PET/SPECT positive disease appears to be resistant to traditional treatment with ^{131}I. Wang et al. reported a series of 25 patients with FDG-avid disease, all of whom received at least one dose of ^{131}I [56]. At follow up the median volume of disease, SUVs and serum Tg had all increased in comparison to a non-randomized control group. Thus, information provided by this diagnostic test may aid in guiding therapy or selecting patients for clinical trials.

Current American Thyroid Association (ATA) guidelines support the consideration of FDG PET/SPECT in patients with elevated Tg and negative RAI scans (grade C) [1]. In addition, these guidelines acknowledge potential emerging roles in a number of other areas that include the following: (i) as a prognostic tool in distant metastatic disease; (ii) selecting patients unlikely to respond to traditional RAI; and (iii) measuring outcomes of other local or systemic therapies.

The role of cross-sectional imaging is less clear and typically guided by symptoms. [1] Chest CT scans or plain radiographs may reveal anatomical evidence of lung metastases. Cross-sectional imaging may be used to confirm rare brain metastases when suggested by symptoms or extensive disease at other sites. Also, traditional ^{99m}Tc bone scintigraphy has a sensitivity approaching 80 % for the detection of bone metastases [50]. However, in the setting of FDG PET/SPECT it is probably redundant, given that PET has a similar sensitivity (85 %) and superior specificity (99 % vs. 91 %) for the detection of bone metastases in these patients [50].

In summary, in 5–45 % of patients that develop distant disease, metastases are evident at the time of diagnosis on cross-sectional imaging or post-therapy RAI scans. The remainder will have distant disease detected during follow-up. In patients with an elevated serum Tg and no evidence of regional disease a search for distant metastases may include diagnostic whole-body RAI scanning. Those patients with elevated Tg and negative scans present a clinical dilemma. More recently, FDG PET/SPECT has shown promise as a diagnostic tool in these patients. The role of FDG PET/SPECT in metastatic thyroid cancer will continue to evolve as more data become available.

Management of Distant Metastases

Given the broad range of outcomes in distant metastatic disease, management of these patients requires multidisciplinary care. Treatment plans may need to be tailored on a case-by-case basis after consideration of factors related to the patient, tumour and subsequently modified according to the response to treatment. Given the relative rarity of metastatic disease in DTC, guidance from large randomized control trials is lacking. As such, management guidelines must derive recommendations from smaller trials, cohort studies and case series. Interestingly, despite the considerable heterogeneity in this patient population, the initial mainstays of treatment are similar and include the following: (i) TSH (thyroid-stimulating hormone or thyrotrophin) suppression; (ii) RAI; and (iii) surgery [1].

TSH Suppression

TSH stimulates thyroid cell proliferation and thus has long been hypothesized to play a potential role in thyroid cancer recurrence. Consequently, TSH suppression with levothyroxine in doses above those required for 'replacement' has been proposed in the management of thyroid cancer. While some conflicting evidence exists, larger studies and meta-analyses have been able to demontrate a link between TSH and a reduction in adverse outcomes [1]. In a study of 2036 patients registered in a multi-institutional thyroid cancer registry, Jonklaas et al. demonstrated improved overall survival in patients with stage II, III or IV disease [4]. Interestingly, whereas a dose-response relationship with the level of TSH suppression was observed in those with more advanced disease (stages III and IV), suppression of the TSH beyond the initial subnormal range in stage II disease did not produce a further incremental benefit. Currently, the ATA recommends aggressive suppression of TSH (<0.1 mU/L) in people with persistent disease but a more conservative approach in those with high-risk (0.1–0.5 mU/L) and low-risk (0.3–2 mU/L) disease in order to prevent recurrence [1]. Clearly, the benefit derived from TSH suppression must be balanced against the potential detrimental effects on cardiac and bone health in each patient.

Radioactive Iodine

RAI ablation following surgery is frequently employed in the primary treatment of DTC. Potential benefits include: (i) facilitating cancer surveillance with serum Tg by ablation of remnant thyroid tissue; (ii) potential reduction in risk of recurrence/disease-specific mortality; and (iii) identification and treatment of persistent disease [1]. When persistent/recurrent metastatic disease is identified, RAI is usually the preferred initial treatment as long as the disease remains iodine-avid [1, 7, 12, 18, 22, 30, 31, 33, 34, 58–61]. The published data on this topic, whereas largely retrospective, does suggest that RAI is of utility in guiding prognosis and might confer a survival benefit.

In addition to iodine avidity, a number of other factors appear predictive of the response to RAI. Durante et al. published a series of 444 patients with distant metastatic disease from PTC or FTC [18]. Of these, 295 were found to have iodine-avid metastatic disease. All patients were treated empirically with 100 mCi. In the setting of persistent iodine-avid disease, treatments were then repeated at 3–12-month intervals until negative studies were obtained. No fixed limit on maximum cumulative dose was set. Overall, 127 patients achieved negative imaging studies during follow-up. A large proportion of these occurred later in the course of therapy (>5 years). In this subset of patients, 10-year survival was 92 % compared to 29 % in those with iodine-avid disease and persistently positive imaging. The 10-year survival of patients without ^{131}I at the outset was just 10 %. The authors examined the characteristics of patients in the most favourable group and found that they were more likely to be young, (<40 years) with PTC, and pulmonary site-only metastases with no findings or micronodular disease on cross-sectional imaging [18]. A number of additional studies have published similar findings supporting the benefit of RAI [6, 7, 10, 15, 22, 34, 58, 61].

Although not universal' most studies seem to indicate that pulmonary disease responds more favourably to RAI than metastases at other sites [7, 15, 18, 22, 36, 61]. Most studies show that the rate of RAI avidity (~67 %) is similar between lung and bone metastases. However' bone metastases appear to be more advanced at the time of diagnosis as most are visible on plain radiographs or cross-sectional imaging [18, 36]. Thus' it would be more reasonable to expect outcomes comparable to those seen in macronodular pulmonary disease. In these subsets' evidence continues to suggest a survival benefit associated with RAI treatment but complete responses are rare [10, 13, 17, 18, 22, 23, 33, 35, 59–61]. As a result' additional therapies play a larger role in the treatment of bone disease.

Current recommendations strongly support the use of RAI in patients with micronodular, iodine-avid disease. In these patients repeated doses should be given at 6–12 month intervals while the disease continues to concentrate iodine and until negative results are achieved [1]. In addition macronodular pulmonary and bone disease may be treated as long as objective benefits are observed [1]. A single safe dose limit has not been defined and the decision to terminate RAI treatment should be individualized to the patient.

The use of therapeutic dose RAI in patients with non-avid disease on diagnostic scans has been an area of considerable controversy. A number of studies have been able to demonstrate an increased sensitivity of post-therapeutic (>100 mCi) whole-body scans compared to diagnostic (<6 mCi) studies [37, 40–42, 48]. Pacini et al. demonstrated uptake on 30/42 post-therapeutic scans in this clinical setting [42]. Those 30 patients were given additional RAI treatments. A mean of three treatments per patient were administered (cumulative range of doses 90–500 mCi) over a period of 6.7 years. Unfortunately' when compared to an untreated group of 28 similar patients' no significant difference in Tg levels or clinical outcomes were observed. More recently' a systematic review published by Ma et al. concluded that insufficient evidence existed to support this approach [40]. Consistent with this assertion' the updated ATA guidelines do not recommend the use of RAI in these groups [1].

The positive outcomes associated with RAI in appropriate patients and the lack of efficacy seen with other treatments for metastatic disease have led to interest in agents that might enhance iodine uptake and retention in non-avid tumours [12, 43–47, 62, 63] Impaired iodine (^{131}I) uptake appears to be related to diminished cell membrane expression of the sodium-iodide symporter. Retinoic acid' via its binding to the retinoic acid receptor' regulates transcription of genes related to cell differentiation. In vitro studies demonstrate some extent of redifferentiation with these compounds [64, 65]. As a result, cells increase their expression of the symporter and take up iodine more efficiently. Unfortunately, clinical studies have failed to show clinical benefit consistently. Courbon et al. reported a series of 11 patients with metastatic DTC and no uptake on whole-body scans [43]. All were treated with 13-cis-retinoic acid. RAI uptake, a surrogate clinical marker of redifferentiation, increased marginally in merely 2 patients. After a mean follow-up of 24 months, 5 patients had died, 5 showed evidence of progression and only one had stable disease. Zhang et al. used another isomer—all-trans-retinoic acid—in 11 patients with advanced-stage DTC and poor RAI uptake [47]. Increase in RAI uptake was seen in 4 patients and diminished uptake in 6. Partial responses were observed in 5 patients and progressive disease was noted in 4 of them. Currently, the use of these compounds outside of a clinical trial cannot be recommended [1].

Lithium has been shown to prolong the duration of RAI uptake by inhibiting its release from the cell [62]. Unfortunately, this effect is not mediated through increase in sodium-iodide symporter expression and thus is only of potential benefit in tumours that are already iodine-avid. Rosiglitazone, a thiazolinedione drug used in patients with diabetes, has shown some early promise in thyroid cancer redifferentiation [44–46]. Rosiglitazone is a peroxisome proliferator-activated receptor gamma agonist. This transcription factor is a regulator of cellular differentiation and has been shown to inhibit tumour development in animal models and human tissue cell lines. Phase II studies have demonstrated some efficacy in increasing RAI uptake in patients with metastatic DTC and negative whole-body scans [44]. Kebebew et al. reported the clinical results of rosiglitazone in 20 patients with DTC and negative RAI whole-body scans [45]. Five patients demonstrated an increase in RAI uptake after treatment. A reduction in Tg level post-therapy was seen in 3 patients. None had a partial response by RECIST criteria and 7 had progressive disease. Thus, whereas this drug shows promise with respect to tumour redifferentiation and increased RAI uptake, significant clinical benefit has yet to be demonstrated. Finally, gene therapy with the introduction of the sodium-iodide symporter gene into tumour cells using an adenovirus vector has been investigated, but its efficacy seems to be limited by short duration of action [63, 66].

The benefits of RAI in the treatment of metastatic DTC must be weighed against potential adverse outcomes. Side-effects typically are related to areas in which the RAI is retained. These include damage to the salivary glands (with risk of dental caries), pulmonary fibrosis in those with diffuse pulmonary disease and second primary cancers. Large epidemiological studies in both Europe and North America have supported an increase in secondary primary cancers with RAI [67–70]. Brown et al. reported an increased risk of second primary cancers with an observed to expected (O/E) ratio of 1:20 in irradiated DTC patients [67]. This risk was greatest in young patients and during the first 5 years after treatment. A dose-response relationship appears to be seen with the cumulative dose of RAI. Thus, no absolute safe dose can be defined but several authors have suggested 600 mCi as a general guideline for clinicians to reconsider the risk: benefit ratio of further therapy.

Surgery

Whereas surgery is a mainstay of treatment in locoregional disease, its application to metastatic disease is more selective. This secondary role is a result of the reality that surgery alone is unlikely to render the patient disease-free. When possible, however, complete surgical extirpation of metastatic disease has been associated with improved survival. Bernier et al. reported a series of 109 of 1977 total DTC patients that developed bone metastases [33]. Of these 109 patients, complete surgical removal of boneonly disease was achieved in 24 and was associated with improved survival. Similar findings were reported in Zettinig et al. in 12 patients in whom complete removal of metastatic bone disease was achieved [23]. In addition, Porterfield et al. reported a series of 48 patients undergoing thoracic metastectomy for DTC metastases [71]. Complete resection was achieved in 69 % and the 10-year overall survival was 60 %. In an earlier study of 16 patients undergoing surgery for lung metastases, the reported 5-year survival was 32 % [72].

In most patients complete surgical removal of all metastatic disease is not possible. The focus of surgical therapy is, therefore, more appropriately directed toward relief of symptoms and prevention of complications. In patients with bone metastases, surgery (along with external beam radiation) plays an important role not only in the palliation of pain, but also in the prevention of complications. Pittas et al. reported on a review of 146 patients with bone metastases and found that 27 % developed a pathological fracture and 14 % suffered neurological compromise [35].

One specific caveat to the relegation of surgery to second-line therapy in distant disease is in the case of cerebral metastases. The efficacy of RAI is questionable and the required elevation of TSH, via levothyroxine withdrawal, may lead to growth and neurological compromise. As such, surgery and external beam radiation have been adopted as the mainstays. of therapy in this group of patients with an admittedly poor prognosis. Chiu et al. reported on a single institution, retrospective series of 47 cases of thyroid cancer with brain metastases [73]. The median survival was significantly longer for those who underwent resection (16.7 months) compared to those who did not (3.4 months). A survival benefit was not seen for any other therapy. If cerebral metastases are unresectable and concentrate RAI, this therapy can be used, but prior radiation and corticosteroids are recommended to ameliorate the potential risks [1].

Thyroid cancer metastasis to unusual sites is typically a marker of disseminated disease. As such, surgery is most frequently aimed at palliation. Small studies reporting resection of thyroid cancer metastases to the skin, adrenal glands and gastrointestinal tract have been published [27, 28, 74, 75]. Given the rarity of this clinical entity, no data suggesting a survival benefit exist. Surgical decision-making in these patients is most appropriately done on a case-by-case basis with the focus on palliation.

Cytotoxic Chemotherapy

Metastatic disease that is both unresponsive to RAI and unresectable presents a major clinical challenge. In general, other therapies have proven disappointing. Systemic therapy with tradition cytotoxic chemotherapy is largely ineffective [76–81]. Single-agent therapy with doxorubicin has been the most commonly studied. In general, partial response rates of 15–30 % have been observed with no complete responses and short duration [77–80]. Combination chemotherapy, with the addition of cisplatin or bleomycin and vincristine, has also been evaluated in small numbers of patients [76, 79–81]. In general, slight increases in response rates with a few complete responses have been observed. However, this small benefit must be balanced against the increase in drug toxicities with fatal events in some patients. Current recommendations allow for a role in patients with extensive disease who are not amenable to more effective therapies, but suggest that the patient may benefit more from entry into a clinical trial of newer molecular therapies if they qualify [1].

External Beam Radiation

The majority of experience with external beam radiation in DTC is in patients with persistent or unresectable locoregional disease. In patients with a residual tumour after surgical resection, external beam radiation has been associated with a reduction in the risk of recurrence [1, 12, 82]. In contrast, data are scant with respect to its use in metastatic DTC. Given the typically diffuse pattern of disease and risk of pulmonary fibrosis, external beam radiation is rarely used in the treatment of lung metastases [1, 82]. One caveat may be in the case of a large localized deposit causing symptoms, such as haemoptysis. External beam radiation has been used for palliation in painful bone metastases or to prevent neurological compromise or pathological fractures in tumours at dangerous locations. Evidence from small series supports the use of external beam radiation alone or in combination with RAI for symptom relief in painful bone metastases [23, 33, 35, 82]. Other therapies for palliation of bone disease, including bisphosphonate infusion and embolization in combination with radiation and/or surgery, may provide additional benefit in the treatment of these patients [83, 84]. Finally, external beam radiation has also been used for unresectable brain metastases, although no evidence of a survival benefit exists in this setting [73].

Molecular Therapies

Given the limited success of traditional systemic therapies in those with disease resistant to traditional thyroid cancer therapies, interest in newer molecular-based therapies for metastatic DTC has been significant. Increasing knowledge of mutations and molecular pathways involved in tumorigenesis and predictive of more aggressive disease has led to the development of precise treatments designed to specifically target critical molecules/pathways. The majority of recent research in this area has focused on tyrosine kinase inhibitors that inhibit multiple pathways typically involved in vascular proliferation, including vascular endothelial growth factor and platelet-derived growth factor. Multiple phase II trials have been completed [85–87]. Whereas partial responses by RECIST criteria have been observed in a number of patients, the enthusiasm has been somewhat tempered by a significant rate of adverse events. The molecular pathways, results of specific trials, and additional potential agents will be discussed in more detail in a subsequent chapter.

Conclusions

Despite the overall excellent prognosis typically associated with DTC, 6–20 % of patients will ultimately develop metastatic disease. In these patients the overall 10-year survival is reported to be 40 %. However, this figure does not reflect the heterogeneity of outcomes in these patients. Young patients with RAI-avid, lung-only micronodular disease that responds to therapy may have 10-year survival rates that exceed 90 %. In contrast, older patients with multiple metastatic sites of RAI-resistant disease have a dismal prognosis. The mainstays of therapy include RAI, TSH suppression, and surgery in select cases. Patients with disease that is resistant to traditional therapies have dismal outcomes with systemic cytotoxic chemotherapy and should be considered for clinical trials into newer molecular agents. Care of these patients should be multidisciplinary in nature and the goals should be individualized to the patient and to the disease.

Commentary

Richard W. Nason

Well-differentiated thyroid cancer (WDTC) has a prolonged natural history and a relatively low mortality rate. Recurrence rates approximate 20 % and are most frequently identified in the neck, followed by distant metastases. The most frequent sites of distant metastases are lung and bone. The overall mortality rate for WDTC in North America approximates 10 %. Disease-specific mortality is distributed between local recurrence and distant metastases. The surgeon has some control over the first cause of morbidity and mortality with an adequate initial operation. As emphasized years ago by Dr Crile, the battle of the thyroid is won or lost in the central compartment. Unfortunately, we have less control over this disease in the presence of distant metastases.

As detailed in this chapter, long-term surveillance of patients with WDTC is important to identify both locoregional recurrence and distant metastases. It should be emphasized that follow-up, in my opinion, needs to be directed to the central compartment, as viable treatment options are often available. As indicated in this chapter, young patients with micronodular radioactive iodine (RAI) avid pulmonary metastases do well with treatment. In my experience, older patients with distant metastases are not cured and this does represent a significant source of morbidity and mortality. In our centre, RAI is the treatment if the disease is radio-avid. An important aspect of care in this subset of patients is clinical follow-up with active assessment of symptoms and signs of bone metastases with effective intervention with surgery with or without external beam radiation to minimize pathological fractures or neurological compromise.

The management of patients with distant metastases from WDTC must be individualized and should be based on the circumstances and the experience of a multidisciplinary treatment team. The future for this subset of patients will lie in the development of effective and personalized systemic treatment, as discussed elsewhere in this monograph.

References

1. American Thyroid Association (ATA) Guidelines Taskforce on Thyroid Nodules and Differentiated Thyroid Cancer, Cooper DS, Doherty GM, Haugen BR, et al. Revised American Thyroid Association management guidelines for patients with thyroid nodules and differentiated thyroid cancer. Thyroid. 2009;19:1167–214.
2. Eustatia-Rutten CF, Corssmit EP, Biermasz NR, et al. Survival and death causes in differentiated thyroid carcinoma. J Clin Endocrinol Metab. 2006;91:313–9.
3. Hundahl SA, Fleming ID, Fremgen AM, et al. A national cancer database report on 53,856 cases of thyroid carcinoma treated in the US, 1985–1995. Cancer. 1998;83:2638–48.
4. Jonklaas J, Sarlis NJ, Litofsky D, et al. Outcomes of patients with differentiated thyroid carcinoma following initial therapy. Thyroid. 2006;16:1229–42.
5. McConahey WM, Hay ID, Woolner LB, et al. Papillary thyroid cancer treated at the Mayo Clinic, 1946 through 1970: initial manifestations, pathologic findings, therapy, and outcome. Mayo Clin Proc. 1986;61:978–96.
6. Benbassat CA, Mechlis-Frish S, Hirsch D. Clinicopathological characteristics and long-term outcome in patients with distant metastases from differentiated thyroid cancer. World J Surg. 2006;30:1088–95.
7. Casara D, Rubello D, Saladini G, et al. Distant metastases in differentiated thyroid cancer: long-term results of radioiodine treatment and statistical analysis of prognostic factors in 214 patients. Tumori. 1991;77:432–6.
8. Clark JR, Lai P, Hall F, et al. Variables predicting distant metastases in thyroid cancer. Laryngoscope. 2005;115:661–7.
9. Hoie J, Stenwig AE, Kullmann G, et al. Distant metastases in papillary thyroid cancer. A review of 91 patients. Cancer. 1988;61:1–6.
10. Lin JD, Huang MJ, Juang JH, et al. Factors related to the survival of papillary and follicular thyroid carcinoma patients with distant metastases. Thyroid. 1999;9:1227–35.
11. Machens A, Holzhausen HJ, Lautenschlager C, et al. Enhancement of lymph node metastasis and distant metastasis of thyroid carcinoma. Cancer. 2003;98:712–9.
12. O'Neill CJ, Oucharek J, Learoyd D, et al. Standard and emerging therapies for metastatic differentiated thyroid cancer. Oncologist. 2010;15:146–56.
13. Ruegemer JJ, Hay ID, Bergstralh EJ, et al. Distant metastases in differentiated thyroid carcinoma: a multivariate analysis of prognostic variables. J Clin Endocrinol Metab. 1988;67:501–8.
14. Samaan NA, Schultz PN, Haynie TP, et al. Pulmonary metastasis of differentiated thyroid carcinoma: treatment results in 101 patients. J Clin Endocrinol Metab. 1985;60:376–80.
15. Sampson E, Brierley JD, Le LW, et al. Clinical management and outcome of papillary and follicular (differentiated) thyroid cancer presenting with distant metastasis at diagnosis. Cancer. 2007;110:1451–6.
16. Showalter TN, Siegel BA, Moley JF, et al. Prognostic factors in patients with well-differentiated thyroid cancer presenting with pulmonary metastasis. Cancer Biother Radiopharm. 2008;23:655–9.
17. Casara D, Rubello D, Saladini G, et al. Different features of pulmonary metastases in differentiated thyroid cancer: natural history and multivariate statistical analysis of prognostic variables. J Nucl Med. 1993;34:1626–31.
18. Durante C, Haddy N, Baudin E, et al. Long-term outcome of 444 patients with distant metastases from papillary and follicular thyroid carcinoma: benefits and limits of radioiodine therapy. J Clin Endocrinol Metab. 2006;91:2892–9.
19. Haq M, Harmer C. Differentiated thyroid carcinoma with distant metastases at presentation: prognostic factors and outcome. Clin Endocrinol (Oxf). 2005;63:87–93.
20. Lin JD, Chao TC, Chou SC, et al. Papillary thyroid carcinomas with lung metastases. Thyroid. 2004;14:1091–6.
21. Shaha AR, Ferlito A, Rinaldo A. Distant metastases from thyroid and parathyroid cancer. ORL J Otorhinolaryngol Relat Spec. 2001;63:243–9.

22. Shoup M, Stojadinovic A, Nissan A, et al. Prognostic indicators of outcomes in patients with distant metastases from differentiated thyroid carcinoma. J Am Coll Surg. 2003;197:191–7.

23. Zettinig G, Fueger BJ, Passler C, et al. Long-term follow-up of patients with bone metastases from differentiated thyroid carcinoma—surgery or conventional therapy? Clin Endocrinol (Oxf). 2002;56:377–82.

24. Welch Dinauer CA, Tuttle RM, Robie DK, et al. Clinical features associated with metastasis and recurrence of differentiated thyroid cancer in children, adolescents and young adults. Clin Endocrinol (Oxf). 1998;49:619–28.

25. Beasley NJ, Walfish PG, Witterick I, et al. Cause of death in patients with well-differentiated thyroid carcinoma. Laryngoscope. 2001;111:989–91.

26. Harness JK, McLeod MK, Thompson NW, et al. Deaths due to differentiated thyroid cancer: a 46-year perspective. World J Surg. 1988;12:623–9.

27. Klubo-Gwiezdzinska J, Morowitz D, Van Nostrand D, et al. Metastases of well-differentiated thyroid cancer to the gastrointestinal system. Thyroid. 2010;20:381–7.

28. Lo CY, van Heerden JA, Soreide JA, et al. Adrenalectomy for metastatic disease to the adrenal glands. Br J Surg. 1996;83:528–31.

29. McWilliams RR, Giannini C, Hay ID, et al. Management of brain metastases from thyroid carcinoma: a study of 16 pathologically confirmed cases over 25 years. Cancer. 2003;98:356–62.

30. Hindie E, Melliere D, Lange F, et al. Functioning pulmonary metastases of thyroid cancer: does radioiodine influence the prognosis? Eur J Nucl Med Mol Imaging. 2003;30:974–81.

31. Nixon IJ, Whitcher MM, Palmer FL, et al. The impact of distant metastases at presentation on prognosis in patients with differentiated carcinoma of the thyroid gland. Thyroid. 2012;22:884–9.

32. Kitamura Y, Shimizu K, Nagahama M, et al. Immediate causes of death in thyroid carcinoma: clinicopathological analysis of 161 fatal cases. J Clin Endocrinol Metab. 1999;84:4043–9.

33. Bernier MO, Leenhardt L, Hoang C, et al. Survival and therapeutic modalities in patients with bone metastases of differentiated thyroid carcinomas. J Clin Endocrinol Metab. 2001;86:1568–73.

34. Schlumberger M, Challeton C, De Vathaire F, et al. Radioactive iodine treatment and external radiotherapy for lung and bone metastases from thyroid carcinoma. J Nucl Med. 1996;37:598–605.

35. Pittas AG, Adler M, Fazzari M, et al. Bone metastases from thyroid carcinoma: clinical characteristics and prognostic variables in one hundred forty-six patients. Thyroid. 2000;10:261–8.

36. Toubert ME, Hindie E, Rampin L, et al. Distant metastases of differentiated thyroid cancer: diagnosis, treatment and outcome. Nucl Med Rev Cent East Eur. 2007;10:106–9.

37. Fatourechi V, Hay ID, Mullan BP, et al. Are posttherapy radioiodine scans informative and do they influence subsequent therapy of patients with differentiated thyroid cancer? Thyroid. 2000;10:573–7.

38. Fatourechi V, Hay ID, Javedan H, et al. Lack of impact of radioiodine therapy in Tg-positive, diagnostic whole-body scan-negative patients with follicular cell-derived thyroid cancer. J Clin Endocrinol Metab. 2002;87:1521–6.

39. Galligan JP, Winship J, van Doorn T, et al. A comparison of serum thyroglobulin measurements and whole body ^{131}I scanning in the management of treated differentiated thyroid carcinoma. Aust N Z J Med. 1982;12:248–54.

40. Ma C, Kuang A, Xie J. Radioiodine therapy for differentiated thyroid carcinoma with thyroglobulin positive and radioactive iodine negative metastases. Cochrane Database Syst Rev. 2009;(1):CD006988.

41. Pacini F, Lippi F, Formica N, et al. Therapeutic doses of iodine-131 reveal undiagnosed metastases in thyroid cancer patients with detectable serum thyroglobulin levels. J Nucl Med. 1987;28:1888–91.

42. Pacini F, Agate L, Elisei R, et al. Outcome of differentiated thyroid cancer with detectable serum Tg and negative diagnostic ^{131}I whole body scan: comparison of patients treated with high ^{131}I activities versus untreated patients. J Clin Endocrinol Metab. 2001;86:4092–7.

43. Courbon F, Zerdoud S, Bastie D, et al. Defective efficacy of retinoic acid treatment in patients with metastatic thyroid carcinoma. Thyroid. 2006;16:1025–31.
44. Kebebew E, Peng M, Reiff E, et al. A phase II trial of rosiglitazone in patients with thyroglobulin-positive and radioiodine-negative differentiated thyroid cancer. Surgery. 2006;140:960–6; discussion 966–7.
45. Kebebew E, Lindsay S, Clark OH, et al. Results of rosiglitazone therapy in patients with thyroglobulin-positive and radioiodine-negative advanced differentiated thyroid cancer. Thyroid. 2009;19:953–6.
46. Tepmongkol S, Keelawat S, Honsawek S, et al. Rosiglitazone effect on radioiodine uptake in thyroid carcinoma patients with high thyroglobulin but negative total body scan: a correlation with the expression of peroxisome proliferator-activated receptor-gamma. Thyroid. 2008;18:697–704.
47. Zhang Y, Jia S, Liu Y, et al. A clinical study of all-trans-retinoid-induced differentiation therapy of advanced thyroid cancer. Nucl Med Commun. 2007;28:251–5.
48. Pineda JD, Lee T, Ain K, et al. Iodine-131 therapy for thyroid cancer patients with elevated thyroglobulin and negative diagnostic scan. J Clin Endocrinol Metab. 1995;80:1488–92.
49. Grunwald F, Schomburg A, Bender H, et al. Fluorine-18 fluorodeoxyglucose positron emission tomography in the follow-up of differentiated thyroid cancer. Eur J Nucl Med. 1996;23:312–9.
50. Ito S, Kato K, Ikeda M, et al. Comparison of 18 F-FDG PET and bone scintigraphy in detection of bone metastases of thyroid cancer. J Nucl Med. 2007;48:889–95.
51. Larson SM, Robbins R. Positron emission tomography in thyroid cancer management. Semin Roentgenol. 2002;37:169–74.
52. Nanni C, Rubello D, Fanti S, et al. Role of 18 F-FDG-PET and PET/CT imaging in thyroid cancer. Biomed Pharmacother. 2006;60:409–13.
53. Schluter B, Bohuslavizki KH, Beyer W, et al. Impact of FDG PET on patients with differentiated thyroid cancer who present with elevated thyroglobulin and negative ^{131}I scan. J Nucl Med. 2001;42:71–6.
54. Wang H, Fu HL, Li JN, et al. Comparison of whole-body 18 F-FDG SPECT and post-therapeutic ^{131}I scintigraphy in the detection of metastatic thyroid cancer. Clin Imaging. 2008;32:32–7.
55. Wang W, Macapinlac H, Larson SM, et al. [18 F]-2-fluoro-2-deoxy-D-glucose positron emission tomography localizes residual thyroid cancer in patients with negative diagnostic ^{131}I whole body scans and elevated serum thyroglobulin levels. J Clin Endocrinol Metab. 1999;84:2291–302.
56. Wang W, Larson SM, Tuttle RM, et al. Resistance of [18f]fluorodeoxyglucose-avid metastatic thyroid cancer lesions to treatment with high-dose radioactive iodine. Thyroid. 2001;11:1169–75.
57. Feine U, Lietzenmayer R, Hanke JP, et al. Fluorine-18-FDG and iodine-131-iodide uptake in thyroid cancer. J Nucl Med. 1996;37:1468–72.
58. Coburn M, Teates D, Wanebo HJ. Recurrent thyroid cancer. Role of surgery versus radioactive iodine (^{131}I). Ann Surg. 1994;219:587–93; discussion 593–5.
59. Hindie E, Zanotti-Fregonara P, Keller I, et al. Bone metastases of differentiated thyroid cancer: Impact of early ^{131}I-based detection on outcome. Endocr Relat Cancer. 2007;14:799–807.
60. Ilgan S, Karacalioglu AO, Pabuscu Y, et al. Iodine-131 treatment and high-resolution CT: results in patients with lung metastases from differentiated thyroid carcinoma. Eur J Nucl Med Mol Imaging. 2004;31:825–30.
61. Pacini F, Cetani F, Miccoli P, et al. Outcome of 309 patients with metastatic differentiated thyroid carcinoma treated with radioiodine. World J Surg. 1994;18:600–4.
62. Liu YY, van der Pluijm G, Karperien M, et al. Lithium as adjuvant to radioiodine therapy in differentiated thyroid carcinoma: clinical and in vitro studies. Clin Endocrinol (Oxf). 2006;64:617–24.
63. Spitzweg C, Morris JC. Gene therapy for thyroid cancer: current status and future prospects. Thyroid. 2004;14:424–34.
64. Kurebayashi J, Tanaka K, Otsuki T, et al. All-trans-retinoic acid modulates expression levels of thyroglobulin and cytokines in a new human poorly differentiated papillary thyroid carcinoma cell line, KTC-1. J Clin Endocrinol Metab. 2000;85:2889–96.

65. Schmutzler C, Brtko J, Bienert K, et al. Effects of retinoids and role of retinoic acid receptors in human thyroid carcinomas and cell lines derived therefrom. Exp Clin Endocrinol Diabetes. 1996;104 Suppl 4:16–9.
66. Boland A, Ricard M, Opolon P, et al. Adenovirus-mediated transfer of the thyroid sodium/iodide symporter gene into tumors for a targeted radiotherapy. Cancer Res. 2000;60:3484–92.
67. Brown AP, Chen J, Hitchcock YJ, et al. The risk of second primary malignancies up to three decades after the treatment of differentiated thyroid cancer. J Clin Endocrinol Metab. 2008;93:504–15.
68. Rubino C, de Vathaire F, Dottorini ME, et al. Second primary malignancies in thyroid cancer patients. Br J Cancer. 2003;89:1638–44.
69. Sawka AM, Thabane L, Parlea L, et al. Second primary malignancy risk after radioactive iodine treatment for thyroid cancer: a systematic review and metaanalysis. Thyroid. 2009;19:451–7.
70. Subramanian S, Goldstein DP, Parlea L, et al. Second primary malignancy risk in thyroid cancer survivors: a systematic review and meta-analysis. Thyroid. 2007;17:1277–88.
71. Porterfield JR, Cassivi SD, Wigle DA, et al. Thoracic metastasectomy for thyroid malignancies. Eur J Cardiothorac Surg. 2009;36:155–8.
72. Protopapas AD, Nicholson AG, Vini L, et al. Thoracic metastasectomy in thyroid malignancies. Ann Thorac Surg. 2001;72:1906–8.
73. Chiu AC, Delpassand ES, Sherman SI. Prognosis and treatment of brain metastases in thyroid carcinoma. J Clin Endocrinol Metab. 1997;82:3637–42.
74. Dahl PR, Brodland DG, Goellner JR, et al. Thyroid carcinoma metastatic to the skin: a cutaneous manifestation of a widely disseminated malignancy. J Am Acad Dermatol. 1997;36:531–7.
75. Koutkia P, Safer JD. Adrenal metastasis secondary to papillary thyroid carcinoma. Thyroid. 2001;11:1077–9.
76. Bukowski RM, Brown L, Weick JK, et al. Combination chemotherapy of metastatic thyroid cancer. Phase II study. Am J Clin Oncol. 1983;6:579–81.
77. Gottlieb JA, Hill Jr CS, Ibanez ML, et al. Chemotherapy of thyroid cancer. An evaluation of experience with 37 patients. Cancer. 1972;30:848–53.
78. Gottlieb JA, Hill Jr CS. Chemotherapy of thyroid cancer with adriamycin. Experience with 30 patients. N Engl J Med. 1974;290:193–7.
79. Hoskin PJ, Harmer C. Chemotherapy for thyroid cancer. Radiother Oncol. 1987;10:187–94.
80. Shimaoka K, Schoenfeld DA, DeWys WD, et al. A randomized trial of doxorubicin versus doxorubicin plus cisplatin in patients with advanced thyroid carcinoma. Cancer. 1985;56:2155–60.
81. Williams SD, Birch R, Einhorn LH. Phase II evaluation of doxorubicin plus cisplatin in advanced thyroid cancer: a Southeastern Cancer Study Group Trial. Cancer Treat Rep. 1986;70:405–7.
82. Ford D, Giridharan S, McConkey C, et al. External beam radiotherapy in the management of differentiated thyroid cancer. Clin Oncol (R Coll Radiol). 2003;15:337–41.
83. Eustatia-Rutten CF, Romijn JA, Guijt MJ, et al. Outcome of palliative embolization of bone metastases in differentiated thyroid carcinoma. J Clin Endocrinol Metab. 2003;88:3184–9.
84. Vitale G, Fonderico F, Martignetti A, et al. Pamidronate improves the quality of life and induces clinical remission of bone metastases in patients with thyroid cancer. Br J Cancer. 2001;84:1586–90.
85. Gupta-Abramson V, Troxel AB, Nellore A, et al. Phase II trial of sorafenib in advanced thyroid cancer. J Clin Oncol. 2008;26:4714–9.
86. Kloos RT, Ringel MD, Knopp MV, et al. Phase II trial of sorafenib in metastatic thyroid cancer. J Clin Oncol. 2009;27:1675–84.
87. Pennell NA, Daniels GH, Haddad RI, et al. A phase II study of gefitinib in patients with advanced thyroid cancer. Thyroid. 2008;18:317–23.

Erik S. Venos and Vicky M. Parkins

Introduction

The development of the American Thyroid Association (ATA) guidelines in 2009 was an important advance in the management of thyroid nodules and well-differentiated thyroid cancer (WDTC) [1]. WDTC is unique among cancers in that while the prevalence is increasing (56,140 estimated new cases diagnosed in the USA in 2012) [2], the outcome for most patients is reasonably good [3]. WDTC can be viewed as a chronic illness similar to diabetes or hypertension, in which patient management is guided essentially by estimation of the risk of survival and disease recurrence vis-a-vis the side-effects and burden of treatment and follow-up.

Consistent with this idea is the development of a 'risk-adapted' paradigm in the management and follow-up of WDTC, in which improved identification of patients at higher or lower risk permits clinicians to undertake the following: (i) better patient management, (ii) dictate follow-up monitoring, and (iii) improve medical and/or surgical management after the initial surgery [4, 5].

The present chapter aims to describe some of these concepts with an emphasis on studies published since the release of the 2009 ATA guidelines, which highlight some of the potential current applications of this risk-adapted paradigm. Particular mention will be made of the controversies relating to completion thyroidectomy, radioactive iodine (RAI) use and preparation, as well as the nuances of management when lymph node are involved. This review focuses on the post-surgical management of WDTC after completion of the initial surgical procedure. Surgical management is covered elsewhere in this monograph. Forms of thyroid cancer not arising

E.S. Venos (✉) • V.M. Parkins
Division of Endocrinology and Metabolism, Department of Medicine, University of Calgary and Alberta Health Services, 1820 Richmond Road SW, Calgary, AB T2T 5C7, Canada
e-mail: Erik.venos@albertahealthservices.ca; Vicky.parkins@albertahealthservices.ca

© K. Alok Pathak, Richard W. Nason, Janice L. Pasieka, Rehan Kazi, Raghav C. Dwivedi 2015
Springer India/Byword Books
K.A. Pathak et al. (eds.), *Management of Thyroid Cancer: Special Considerations*, Head and Neck Cancer Clinics, DOI 10.1007/978-81-322-2434-1_7

from the follicular cell (anaplastic thyroid cancer, lymphoma and medullary thyroid cancer) are not discussed.

Initial Assessment of Risk: WDTC Staging

The first step in post-surgical management of WDTC is the appropriate staging of the patient once complete surgical and pathological data are available. As with other solid-organ tumours, the American Joint Committee on Cancer (AJCC) is the standard accepted method of initial staging of a patient with WDTC [6]. In order to comply with convention, tumour size (T), nodal status (N) and metastasis (M) have been defined for thyroid cancer. In brief, T1 are tumours of <2 cm, T2 are between 2 and 4 cm and T3 are >4 cm or have minimal extrathyroidal extension [6]. The latest iteration of the AJCC has T1 broken into Tla (<1 cm) and T2b (1–2 cm). An additional 'm' designation allows for the description of multifocal thyroid tumours. Finally, T4 tumours are divided by the degree of invasion into surrounding structures: T4a is invasion into proximal structures whereas T4b is defined by the invasion into prevertebral fascia, carotid or mediastinal vessels. Lymph node involvement is divided into no lymph nodes (N0), N1a if level VI nodes are involved, and N1b if other cervical or mediastinal nodes are present. Finally, metastases are either absent (M0) or present (M1) [6]. Unlike other solid-organ tumours, age also has a significant impact on mortality owing to differences in response to therapy and inherent tumour biology [7]. Hence, patients <45 years of age at diagnosis are divided by the presence of metastasis alone (M0 – stage I vs. M1 – stage II). On the other hand, patients >45 years of age at the time of diagnosis have staging with progressively increasing risk of mortality from stage I to stage IV [7]. Despite its most recent revision, the staging of WDTC has remained relatively stable over several decades. This is particularly relevant to slowly progressive Amours, which occur in the majority of WDTC.

It is important to note that TNM staging is based on mortality data and, as such, is more relevant to rapidly progressing tumours. However, the majority of WDTC tumours are slow-growing and the main clinical concern is not so much mortality but recurrence and the morbidity associated with those recurrences, be it locoregional or metastatic. Many different adjunctive staging systems have been developed, each of which has been validated separately. Lang and colleagues have compared staging systems in terms of efficacy [8]. The scoring system that is employed most commonly is the metastasis, age, completeness of resection, invasion, size of primary tumour (MACIS) score, as it is calculated using readily available parameters and is predictive of disease-specific death [9]. However, these scoring/risk systems are still routed in mortality data.

As the more frequent clinical problem is that of disease recurrence, the goal is to better predict the risk of disease recurrence. Given the general congruence between factors that affect mortality and those that predict recurrence, a patient with a high risk of death from disease also has a high risk of recurrent disease. The recent ATA staging system for risk of recurrence has added a temporal dimension to patient follow-up [3]. The inherent notion is that response to initial therapy is linked intimately with risk of recurrence. On this basis patients are divided broadly into the following categories: (i) low-, (ii) intermediate-and (iii) high-risk of recurrence. These categories are based on readily available clinical data postoperatively, similar to the information required for postoperative staging (e.g., MACIS).

In this way, the higher risk variants of papillary thyroid carcinoma (PTC), such as tall cell, sclerosing and columnar, as well as Hurthle and follicular carcinoma, are already identified as behaving more aggressively than their TMN staging would dictate. Low-risk features are no local or distant disease, no vascular/local invasion, and no high-risk histologies. Intermediate risk features would include high-risk histologies, microscopic extrathyroidal invasion into vasculature or local structures, and cervical lymph node involvement. High-risk features would include gross invasion, gross postoperative residual disease, and distant metastasis. Response to therapy is evaluated over 2 years of follow-up with usual clinical criteria (thyroglobulin [Tg], neck ultrasonography with or without cross-sectional imaging) and secondary risk stratification is subsequently performed. From here on, based on initial risk estimates of recurrence and subsequent response to therapy, the patient can go on to a rational long-term follow-up strategy commensurate with their risk of morbidity and recurrence from WDTC, as suggested by Tuttle and Leboeuf [4].

For the majority of patients with WDTC, there is rarely a need to escalate therapy as most patients respond well to initial treatment (surgery with or without RAI). This new paradigm of treatment allows for patient individualization and better tailors treatment to risk from disease. If a patient is 'low risk' for mortality and morbidity, a conservative management strategy will suffice. However, it is important to note that these paradigms generally apply to patients at lower risk and not to patients with metastatic disease at presentation, for which their outcomes are generally much worse. Nixon and colleagues recently reviewed the outcomes of patients with metastatic disease at the time of diagnosis of WDTC, a group consisting of 2.9 % of the total cohort. This group has much worse outcomes with a 5-year overall survival and 5-year disease-free survival of 65 % and 68 %, respectively [10]. For such patients, an aggressive approach involving multiple modalities is more appropriate.

A major drawback of the ATA recurrence risk system is the characteristics surrounding the initial remnant ablation/treatment with RAI and reliance on Tg as a tumour marker. This will not apply necessarily to those patients who did not receive RAI. A more recent scoring system for risk of recurrence has been developed on the basis of papillary microcarcinoma. The study by Buffet and colleagues shows a higher recurrence in male patients, multifocal tumours and minimal extrathyroidal extension. This scoring system may help guide management for these low-risk tumours in the future [11].

Completion Thyroidectomy in Incidentally Discovered WDTC

The finding of incidental WDTC is common. Roti et al. [12], in a systematic review on the subject, found that the autopsy rate of thyroid microcarcinoma varied from 0.01 % in the USA to 35.6 % in Finland. The incidental prevalence also varies. For benign thyroid disease, the prevalence ranged from 3.1 to 21 % [12]. In multinodular goitre, the range of incidental thyroid cancer has been found to be 3.1–15.2 % [12]. These findings present a problem for both endocrine surgeons and endocrinologists when patients are found to have incidental PTC, especially when a hemithyroidectomy is performed for an otherwise benign lesion, for example in Graves disease or a toxic nodule. Options available to the treating team would be to observe, perform a completion hemithyroidectomy, or treatment with RAI.

For incidental thyroid cancer, the ATA guidelines recommend completion thyroidectomy for those patients for whom a total or neartotal thyroidectomy would have been recommended had the diagnosis been available before surgery [1]. An exception is made for small (<1 cm), unifocal, intrathyroidal, N0, low-risk Amours. RAI-remnant ablation in this scenario was not recommended. Evidence is strong regarding the presence of contralateral thyroid cancer in the setting of multifocal primary PTC [13]. Lin and Bhattacharyya's study from Boston also supports the fact that lobectomy has the same disease-specific survival for papillary microcarcinoma in an analysis of 7,818 patients from the Surveillance, Epidemiology and End Results (SEER) database [14]. Another area of guidance would be to examine the outcomes of those who had either a lobectomy or total thyroidectomy when the primary cancer is known in advance. The largest study pertaining to this question comes from an analysis of the US National Cancer Database, which indicated that patients with a lobectomy had an increased risk of recurrence (HR 1.15 [1.02–1.30; p=0.04]) and decreased overall survival (HR 1.31 [1.07–1.60; p=0.009]) if the primary tumour was >1 cm [15].

In recent years, the practice of total thyroidectomy for patients with WDTC >1 cm has been questioned, with some authors, using case series from their institutions, arguing that lobectomy may be sufficient for Amours of >1 cm. This becomes particularly relevant if the patient has suffered from a complication during the initial lobectomy procedure. Vaisman and colleagues presented their retrospective case review from one thyroid cancer specialist's practice, which involved 72 patients with lobectomy alone, and compared them to 217 patients with total thyroidectomy, where neither group received RAI [16]. It is pertinent that 55 % of the 289 total patients had primary Amours of >1 cm. The rate of structural recurrence was 2.3 % for complete thyroidectomy and 4.2 % for lobectomy alone over a median of 5 years of follow-up. In all recurrences in the lobectomy group, the patient had no evident disease after completion thyroidectomy and RAI [16]. A larger study was conducted at the same centre on 869 patients with pT1T2 intrathyroidal cancers treated surgically from 1985 to 2005 [17]. Total thyroidectomy was performed in 59 % of patients and thyroid lobectomy was performed in 41 % of patients. Patients were followed for a median of 99 months. In this cohort, the 10-year overall survival, disease-specific survival and recurrence-free survival were 92 %, 99 % and 98 %, respectively. Multivariate analysis showed that age >45 years and male gender were independent risk factors for poorer overall survival whereas T stage and type of surgery were not [17]. It should be noted that total thyroidectomies were performed at this centre in all patients with a nodule in the opposite lobe. Thus, lobectomy alone may be sufficient in certain cases with a larger primary tumour provided there are no clinically involved lymph nodes, a younger age, no nodules in the remaining lobe, and no extrathyroidal extension at initial surgery.

The Risk-Adjusted use of RAI: Selecting the Appropriate Patients While Attempting to Minimize Adverse Effects

Clinicians are able to reassure patients about a good prognosis on the basis of the success of surgical management in an age of increasing prevalence of WDTC. On the other hand, the lack of consensus on the administration of RAI in low-risk patients can leave patients feeling concerned, especially as the absolute benefit to the patient regarding recurrence and overall survival may be small or non-existent. Guidelines on the administration of RAI have become more conservative over time, with strong recommendations on its administration being more limited [1, 18].

The lack of consensus on the optimum use of RAI is manifested by studies across populations that indicate a wide variation in its use. Data from the US National Cancer Database compiled from 1990 to 2008 reveal a few trends [19]. A significant increase was found in the proportion of patients receiving RAI from 1990 to 2008—1373/3397 (40.4 %) in 1990 and 11,539/20,620 (56.0 %) in 2008; $p < 0.001$. Whereas a significant difference was seen between RAI ablation between patients who had stage I versus stage IV thyroid cancer (OR 0.34 [0.31–0.37]), this difference was not evident for other stages of cancer. The authors found that only 21.1 % of variation was based on tumour characteristics, whereas hospital type and case volume accounted for 17.1 % of this difference. Finally, 29.1 % of the difference was attributable to unexplained hospital characteristics.

Despite an increase in the use of RAI, its effectiveness in persons with low-risk thyroid cancer has been questioned. Sacks et al. in a systematic review found 70 studies published since 1966 that compared treatment with no treatment [18]. None of the studies were randomized, with most using a retrospective cohort design. No high quality studies have shown an increase in overall survival with the use of RAI. A 10-year follow-up of two centres in France showed similar findings. Review of data from 1,298 low-risk WDTC patients treated with total thyroidectomy with or without RAI showed no difference in overall survival or disease-free survival [20]. The adverse effects of RAI also need to be weighed when recommending appropriate therapy to patients. One recent area of concern involves the development of secondary cancers, especially as it relates to patients with an otherwise good prognosis. An analysis of the SEER database evaluated trends in the administration of RAI from the years 1973 to 2007 [21]. In this cohort, the use of RAI in patients with low-risk (T1N0) cancer increased from 3.3 to 38.1 %. The excess attributable risk of leukaemia was compared across 8-year time periods with this value increasing from 0.2 excess cases per 10,000 patient-years (1973–1981) to 2 excess cases per 10,000 patient-years (1999–2006). Salivary gland malignancies were also found to be higher in those treated with RAI. The same trend appears from the same SEER database review but from a different group (University of Utah) [22].

RAI Dosing and the Use of THW Compared with rhTSH in Patients at a Low Risk and an Intermediate-High Risk of Recurrence

One possible solution to this problem would be to consider the use of lower doses of RAI, especially for patients with lower risk of thyroid cancer. The standard dose of iodine used for the treatment of thyroid cancer is 100 mCi (3.7 GBq) while a lower dose of RAI is 30 mCi (1.1 GBq). For practitioners who favour the more liberal use of RAI for patients with low-risk thyroid cancer, two recent randomized controlled trials investigated the effects of different doses of RAI and the use of recombinant human thyroid-stimulating hormone (rhTSH), a recombinant form of TSH, compared to thyroid hormone withdrawal (THW) [23, 24].

Mallick and colleagues randomized 440 patients with T1-T3 disease with the possibility of having lymph node involvement but no distant or residual surgical disease in a 2×2 factorial design to low-dose RAI versus high-dose RAI along with randomization to pre-RAI preparation with rhTSH or THW [23]. The primary outcome was a negative Tg or a negative diagnostic scan (when anti-Tg antibodies were positive) at 6–9 months post-treatment. Overall, no difference was seen in treatment success using either RAI dose and using either preparation method. Patients receiving a lower dose of RAI spent less time in hospital and reported fewer adverse effects than those receiving the higher dose.

Schlumberger et al. also assessed the value of low-dose RAI and the rhTSH preparation method with their randomized, phase III trial of 752 patients with low-risk WDTC [24]. There was a similar finding of no difference in recurrence with low-dose RAI or the rhTSH preparation method, using Tg as a marker of recurrence, measured during 6–10 months of follow-up [24]. In response to a letter to the editor on the usefulness of RAI in the treatment of low-risk WDTC as a whole, Schlumberger et al. stated that they were launching a prospective, randomized trial, enrolling patients with small thyroid cancers (≤ 10 mm) and multifocal disease, or solitary cancers from 11 to 20 mm and no lymph-node metastases [25]. This trial would compare outcomes after low-dose radioiodine ablation following the use of rhTSH with no ablation. It is hoped that the investigators are able to recruit a sufficient number of patients, to power the trial adequately to answer this important clinical question.

Whereas these results would give practitioners confidence in using a lower dose of RAI along with rhTSH, the question remains about whether rhTSH could be used for patients with medium to high risk of recurrence, as assessed by the ATA criteria [1]. A recent retrospective review addressed this question by comparing the clinical outcomes of patients at intermediate and high risk of recurrence by the ATA criteria when treated with RAI, prepared by THW versus rhTSH [26]. Overall, no clinical difference was seen in recurrence rates (1.2 % for THW vs. 1.5 % for rhTSH), the likelihood of having persistent disease (48 % for THW vs. 46 % for rhTSH), or the likelihood of having no evidence of disease (52 % for THW vs. 53 % for rhTSH). This finding did not vary across ATA risk groups or AJCC stages. It should be noted that the median dose was more in the conventional range of 109 mCi for THW and

125 mCi for rhTSH [26]. The same group has also found that rhTSH-primed RAI is equally effective in locoregional and pulmonary metastatic disease [27]. This study looked at 84 WDTC patients who had RAI-avid disease outside the thyroid bed at the time of remnant ablation. With similar doses (108 mCi in THW and 144 mCi in rhTSH), the efficacy of elimination of the locoregional disease was 70 % for rhTSH and 63 % for THW (p=0.65). For pulmonary metastases, 3/4 patients with rhTSH and 1/4 patients with THW had no evident disease (p=0.41) after initial RAI treatment [27].

Finally, although the THW method versus the rhTSH method may be considered clinically equivalent, concerns have been expressed from an economic perspective about the extra cost of rhTSH (US $2,000–$8,000) and the need for two additional clinic visits for administration of rhTSH as compared with THW [28]. A cost: utility analysis noted a favourable incremental value with the use of rhTSH [29], On the other hand, another review found a marginal benefit in incremental cost: utility, noting that the model was sensitive to the cost of rhTSH, time off work, and quality of life inputs [30]. The significant benefit of rhTSH in terms of quality of life came from initial studies that evaluated the efficacy of rhTSH [31]. This study by Pacini and colleagues was a multicentre randomized controlled trial showing that patients who underwent RAI treatment had significantly improved SF-36 scores in domains of physical roles and functioning, vitality, social functioning and mental health [31].

The Risk-Adjusted Approach to Locally Advanced Lymph Node Disease, Thyroid Bed Nodules, and Microscopic Extrathyroidal Extension

During follow-up for WDTC, it is not unusual for patients to develop lymph node recurrence. In the past several years the optimal management strategy has been debated. The clinical question relies on the risk of progression to more severe disease from locoregional recurrence. The distinction between whether nodes are detected clinically versus ultrasonographically, the number of nodes present, and the presence of extranodal extension are factors that influence treatment decisions. Randolph and colleagues summarized their review of the literature for cancers classified as pathological N1 [32]. Compared with the median risk of recurrence for clinical N0 cancers (median 2 %, range 0–9 %), there was an increased rate of recurrence for <5 metastatic nodes (median 4 %, range 3–8 %), >5 metastatic nodes (median 19 %, range 7–21 %), clinical N1 (median 22 %, range 10–42 %), and clinical N1 with extranodal extension (median 24 %, range 15–32 %) [32]. This implies that patients who are microscopic N1 with <5 metastatic nodes have almost as low a rate of recurrence as those who have no nodes and, as such, may not need RAI or may require less rigorous postoperative monitoring.

Although Tg and highly sensitive ultrasound have proven value in the monitoring of patients, these modalities also have a greater propensity for revealing residual disease, which may be insignificant, but could also represent recurrence of thyroid cancer. The recurrence rate of PTC in the lateral neck has been found to be at least

15 % [33]. For patients with disease confined to the neck, the 2009 ATA guidelines recommended that therapeutic comprehensive compartmental lateral and/or central neck dissection, which spares uninvolved vital structures, should be performed for patients with persistent or recurrent disease confined to the neck [1]. Lymph nodes of >0.8 cm were considered to be significant. The standard management for such an approach would be biopsy along with central or lateral neck dissection. Reoperation can achieve biochemical · remission, with 27 % of patients ($n = 70$) shown to achieve remission in one series [34]. This series also reported low complication rates from such surgery while acknowledging that the complication rates in earlier series carried ≤20 % morbidity in the form of recurrent laryngeal nerve injury and hypoparathyroidism [35].

A recent study indicates that a more conservative approach should be taken in patients with suspicious cervical nodes detected after thyroidectomy [36]. This retrospective review consisted of 166 patients with abnormal lymph nodes detected on at least two consecutive ultrasounds. The investigators excluded patients who they determined to be at high risk of progression, such as poorly differentiated pathology, markedly PET-positive disease, a history of rapid progression, concern for potential complications from local invasion, lymph nodes >2 cm in size, or multiple 1 cm to 1.5 cm suspicious lymph nodes. The cohort's average age was 41 years (17–80 years) and consisted of 63 % female patients. The ATA initial risk classification stratified 77 % of the cohort at intermediate risk of recurrence. Overall, during a median duration of follow-up of 3.5 years (range 1–13 years), a 3 mm or more increase in lymph node size occurred in 20 % of patients whereas a 5 mm or more enlargement occurred in 9 % of patients [36]. Salvage surgery was felt to be required in 13 % of patients. No local complications related to abnormal lymph nodes of disease-related mortality occurred in the cohort. Of the abnormal lymph node characteristics, only increased vascularity (present in 10 of 15 growing lymph nodes compared to its presence in 50 of 133 nongrowing lymph nodes) was more common (p = 0.04).

The same group had published a similar retrospective review of the natural history of ultrasonographically detected small thyroid bed nodules after total thyroidectomy [37]. This review identified 191 patients with at least one nodule (<11 mm, median size 5 mm) identified after the first postoperative ultrasound. Over a follow-up of 5 years, 9 % of patients (17/191) had an increase in size of one of the nodules. Suspicious features on ultrasound were less useful in predicting which nodules will subsequently grow. Whereas there were 63 % of the nodules detected on initial ultrasound having suspicious features, these features had only a positive predictive value of 0.17. However, the lack of suspicious ultrasound features, absence of cervical lymph nodes and lack of rise of serum Tg all suggest that lack of concerning features in postoperative thyroid bed nodules all but exclude later clinically relevant growth and thus can be monitored in a conservative way.

Whereas gross extrathyroidal extension has been associated with an increased recurrence rate, the question remains as how best to manage pT1/T2N0 patients who have been upstaged to pT3 on the basis of microscopic extrathyroidal extension. In a retrospective comparison of 899 patients with pTl/pT2N0 WDTC compared with 115 patients with WDTC upstaged to pT3 on the basis of microscopic extrathyroidal extension, no difference was seen in 10-year disease-specific survival (99 % vs. 100 %; p=0.733) or recurrence-free survival (98 % vs. 95 %; p=0.188) [38]. The extent of resection and the use of RAI were not found to affect overall outcome [38].

Patient-Centered Approaches to Risk and Using Systems Approaches to Optimize Care

Tying this together, clinicians have looked at the use of decision-aids to assist patients with the decision to undergo RAI ablation, realizing that patients will value the benefits and drawbacks of a proposed treatment differently [39]. In a randomized study of 74 patients with early-stage thyroid cancer after thyroidectomy, the group randomized to the decision-aid arm had improved medical knowledge about PTC and RAI treatment as well as less decisional conflict about the decision (p<0.001). No clear difference between groups was seen in proportion of patients choosing RAI—decision-aid group (11 of 37, 29.7 %) and control group (7 of 37, 18.9 %) [40].

However, these types of approaches are only as good as the information that clinicians have available to assist patients and the communication skills between the various team members. This is important, especially as medical care is becoming increasingly complex and there are an increasing number of providers from which patients can receive their care. Recognizing this, the ATA recently released guidelines on the important preoperative, intraoperative and postoperative information that would allow for optimal patient care [41]. This approach to standardization seems compelling, and it is hoped that it would lead to improved patient outcomes, given that much of the treatment of thyroid cancer is delivered in a community setting [42]. This study is particularly interesting as the bulk of thyroid cancer management is provided outside tertiary thyroid cancer care centres [42].

Future Directions in Assessing Risk

The field of WDTC is evolving constantly. Research into the biology of these tumours is ongoing. The spectrum of disease ascribed to cancers of follicular cell origin is broad and is related to its unique molecular footprint. The occurrence of prototypical genes on these cancers, such as BRAF and RET-PTC, can connote different tumour behaviour [43, 44]. The utility of molecular diagnostics is increasingly important in the characterization of thyroid nodule cytology and is becoming well established [45]. Currently the same molecular testing does not yet play a role in the management of post-surgical thyroid cancer. However, this paradigm exists in many other solid-organ tumours, such as breast cancer and medullary thyroid cancer. In the future, research may define a role for molecular tumour typing in both the prognosis and management of WDTC.

The current treatment paradigm for WDTC after initial surgery and at detection of recurrent disease focuses on further surgery, RAI and external beam radiation. Once these treatments are no longer possible or effective, conventional chemotherapy has been offered, with limited success [1]. The development of the tyrosine kinase inhibitors (TKIs) has ushered a new era of targeted therapy in WDTC when conventional therapies have failed. Currently, many of these drugs are investigational; however, the initial data on these agents appear promising [1, 46]. The future may see an expanded role for TKIs in earlier stage disease if efficacy is achieved without any adverse events.

Conclusions

The authors of this chapter have hoped to show the potential applications of the risk-adapted paradigm to the management of WDTC. In particular, patients who respond to initial therapy and are low-risk can be followed by a conservative strategy. Patients with high-risk disease need to be followed with more aggressive screening using adjunctive modalities, such as cross-sectional imaging (CT, MRI and PET scanning) and considered for more aggressive treatments, including systemic chemotherapy, if progressive disease is evident. Whereas the majority of patients with lower-risk disease and a good response to initial therapy can have a de-escalation of surveillance, the few patients will always remain who require an escalation of surveillance and therapy. The optimal management strategy for an individual patient can be enhanced through development of guidelines encouraging the standardization of perioperative reporting to improve staging and estimation of risk recurrence.

In the past few years, research has helped to broaden the category of patients in whom a more conservative management strategy may be used, thereby exposing patients to fewer complications from treatment that ultimately may not affect outcome. Consideration of the avoidance of completion thyroidectomy in appropriately selected patients with incidentally discovered unifocal WDTC of >1 cm has been demonstrated. Also, the staging system has been refined to consider overall survival and disease-free survival when lymph node disease and local invasiveness are present. Microscopic metastases that number <5 may be classified as a lower risk of recurrence. Patients with microscopic, as opposed to gross, extrathyroidal extension (upstaged to pT3) can show similar clinical outcomes to those with pT1/pT2 disease. Smaller cervical lymph nodes (<1.5 cm) may simply be followed expectantly, as a substantial proportion of these may not progress. Small thyroid bed nodules noted after thyroidectomy may be observed, with negative concerning features on ultrasound helpful in predicting benign nature.

Controversies continue on the use of RAI remnant ablation for patients with low-risk thyroid cancer. This treatment is highly effective for high-risk disease from both a mortality and recurrence perspective. However, use of this method varies across centres for lower risk disease. The equivocal evidence of effectiveness and concern about the risk of secondary malignancies further questions its role in low-risk disease. Promotion of the use of decision-aids to improve patients' medical knowledge and reduce their decisional conflict on whether to undergo RAI is still in its developmental stage. Nevertheless, lower doses of RAI in combination with rhTSH have been shown to have similar outcomes to THW and higher dose RAI in the treatment of low-risk WDTC, as well as patients at intermediate to high risk of recurrence. Ultimately, this allows for less overall radiation exposure.

On the whole, the field of WDTC continues to evolve at an ever-increasing pace. As clinicians, we hope to continue to incorporate this knowledge to best serve the needs of our patients while constantly striving towards improvement [47]. As much of the recommendations are based on reviews from single institutions, where there may be wide variations in the patient population and experience of the practitioner, practitioners should also seek to validate their local practice in comparison to these studies [48]. As always, further studies are necessary, and the publication of experiences, either from single-institution reviews, multi-institution reviews, or from prospective studies, will only serve to bolster clinicians' local practice, as well as the practice of their colleagues as more research-based information becomes available.

Commentary

K. Alok Pathak

Management of well-differentiated thyroid cancer (WTDC) has been based on risk stratification, which in turn is based on various known prognostic factors, such as age, extrathyroidal extension, presence of distant metastasis, etc. While the majority of patients have a low-risk disease and a good response to initial therapy, a few patients require aggressive treatment. In this chapter, Doctors Venos and Parkins demonstrate the potential applications of the risk-adapted paradigm to the management of WDTC. Patients, who respond to initial therapy and are at a low-risk of treatment failure, can be followed by a conservative strategy, whereas those with high-risk disease need to be followed with more aggressive screening for disease progression with anatomical and functional imaging and need to be considered for more aggressive treatments, if required. The cost implications and long-term sequelae of aggressive treatment and intense surveillance need to be balanced against the perceived likely benefit. The authors have discussed at length the American Thyroid Association's stratification system for risk of recurrence, which is one such attempt to develop post-treatment surveillance recommendation for risk-based follow-up.

References

1. American Thyroid Association (ATA) Guidelines Taskforce on Thyroid Nodules and Differentiated Thyroid Cancer, Cooper DS, Doherty GM, Haugen BR, et al. Revised American Thyroid Association management guidelines for patients with thyroid nodules and differentiated thyroid cancer. Thyroid. 2009;19:1167–214.
2. Siegel R, Naishadham D, Jemal A. Cancer statistics, 2012. CA Cancer J Clin. 2012;62:10–29.

3. Tuttle RM, Tala H, Shah J, et al. Estimating risk of recurrence in differentiated thyroid cancer after total thyroidectomy and radioactive iodine remnant ablation: using response to therapy variables to modify the initial risk estimates predicted by the new American Thyroid Association staging system. Thyroid. 2010;20:1341–9.
4. Tuttle RM, Leboeuf R. Follow up approaches in thyroid cancer: a risk adapted paradigm. Endocrinol Metab Clin North Am. 2008;37:419–35.
5. Tuttle RM, Rondeau G, Lee NY. A risk-adapted approach to the use of radioactive iodine and external beam radiation in the treatment of well-differentiated thyroid cancer. Cancer Control. 2011;18:89–95.
6. Greene FL, Page DL, Fleming ID, et al. AJCC cancer staging handbook. 6th ed. New York: Springer; 2002.
7. Jonklaas J, Nogueras-Gonzalez G, Munsell M, et al. The impact of age and gender on papillary thyroid cancer survival. J Clin Endocrinol Metab. 2012;97:E878–87.
8. Lang BH, Lo CY, Chan WF, et al. Staging systems for papillary thyroid carcinoma: a review and comparison. Ann Surg. 2007;245:366–78.
9. Hay ID, Bergstralh EJ, Goellner JR, et al. Predicting outcome in papillary thyroid carcinoma: development of a reliable prognostic scoring system in a cohort of 1779 patients surgically treated at one institution during 1940 through 1989. Surgery. 1993;114:1050–7; discussion 1057–8.
10. Nixon IJ, Whitcher MM, Palmer FL, et al. The impact of distant metastases at presentation on prognosis in patients with differentiated carcinoma of the thyroid gland. Thyroid. 2012;22:884–9.
11. Buffet C, Golmard JL, Hoang C, et al. Scoring system for predicting recurrences in patients with papillary thyroid microcarcinoma. Eur J Endocrinol. 2012;167:267–75.
12. Roti E, degli Uberti EC, Bondanelli M, et al. Thyroid papillary microcarcinoma: a descriptive and meta-analysis study. Eur J Endocrinol. 2008;159:659–73.
13. Pazaitou-Panayiotou K, Capezzone M, Pacini F. Clinical features and therapeutic implication of papillary thyroid microcarcinoma. Thyroid. 2007;17:1085–92.
14. Lin HW, Bhattacharyya N. Survival impact of treatment options for papillary microcarcinoma of the thyroid. Laryngoscope. 2009;119:1983–7.
15. Bilimoria KY, Bentrem DJ, Ko CY, et al. Extent of surgery affects survival for papillary thyroid cancer. Ann Surg. 2007;246:375–84.
16. Vaisman F, Shaha A, Fish S, et al. Initial therapy with either thyroid lobectomy or total thyroidectomy without radioactive iodine remnant ablation is associated with very low rates of structural disease recurrence in properly selected patients with differentiated thyroid cancer. Clin Endocrinol (Oxf). 2011;75:112–9.
17. Nixon IJ, Ganly I, Patel SG, et al. Thyroid lobectomy for treatment of well differentiated intrathyroid malignancy. Surgery. 2012;151:571–9.
18. Sacks W, Fung CH, Chang JT, et al. The effectiveness of radioactive iodine for treatment of low-risk thyroid cancer: a systematic analysis of the peer-reviewed literature from 1966 to April 2008. Thyroid. 2010;20:1235–45.
19. Haymart MR, Banerjee M, Stewart AK, et al. Use of radioactive iodine for thyroid cancer. JAMA. 2011;306:721–8.
20. Schvartz C, Bonnetain F, Dabakuyo S, et al. Impact on overall survival of radioactive iodine in low-risk differentiated thyroid cancer patients. J Clin Endocrinol Metab. 2012;97:1526–35.
21. Iyer NG, Morris LGT, Tuttle RM, et al. Rising incidence of second cancers in patients with low-risk (T1N0) thyroid cancer who receive radioactive iodine therapy. Cancer. 2011;117:4439–46.
22. Brown AP, Chen J, Hitchcock YJ, et al. The risk of second primary malignancies up to three decades after the treatment of differentiated thyroid cancer. J Clin Endocrinol Metab. 2008;93:504–15.
23. Mallick U, Harmer C, Yap B, et al. Ablation with low-dose radioiodine and thyrotropin alfa in thyroid cancer. N Engl J Med. 2012;366:1674–85.
24. Schlumberger M, Catargi B, Borget I, et al. Strategies of radioiodine ablation in patients with low-risk thyroid cancer. N Engl J Med. 2012;366:1663–73.

25. Orlov S, Freeman JL, Walfish PG. Radioiodine ablation in low-risk thyroid cancer. N Engl J Med. 2012;367:672; author reply 673–5.
26. Hugo J, Robenshtok E, Grewal R, et al. Recombinant human thyroid stimulating hormone-assisted radioactive iodine remnant ablation in thyroid cancer patients at intermediate to high risk of recurrence. Thyroid. 2012;22:1007–15.
27. Tuttle RM, Lopez N, Leboeuf R, et al. Radioactive iodine administered for thyroid remnant ablation following recombinant human thyroid stimulating hormone preparation also has an important adjuvant therapy function. Thyroid. 2010;20:257–63.
28. Alexander EK, Larsen PR. Radioiodine for thyroid cancer—is less more? N Engl J Med. 2012;366:1732–3.
29. Mernagh P. Cost-effectiveness of using recombinant human TSH prior to radioiodine ablation for thyroid cancer, compared with treating patients in a hypothyroid state: The German perspective. Eur J Endocrinol. 2006;155:405–14.
30. Wang TS, Cheung K, Mehta P, et al. To stimulate or withdraw? A cost-utility analysis of recombinant human thyrotropin versus thyroxine withdrawal for radioiodine ablation in patients with low-risk differentiated thyroid cancer in the United States. J Clin Endocrinol Metab. 2010;95:1672–80.
31. Pacini F, Ladenson PW, Schlumberger M, et al. Radioiodine ablation of thyroid remnants after preparation with recombinant human thyrotropin in differentiated thyroid carcinoma: results of an international, randomized, controlled study. J Clin Endocrinol Metab. 2006;91:926–32.
32. Randolph G, Duh QY, Heller KS, et al. The prognostic significance of nodal metastases from papillary thyroid carcinoma can be stratified based on the size and number of metastatic lymph nodes, as well as the presence of extranodal extension ATA surgical affairs committee's taskforce on thyroid cancer nodal surgery. Thyroid. 2012;10.
33. Hay ID, Thompson GB, Grant CS, et al. Papillary thyroid carcinoma managed at the mayo clinic during six decades (1940–1999): temporal trends in initial therapy and long-term outcome in 2444 consecutively treated patients. World J Surg. 2002;26:879–85.
34. Al-Saif O, Farrar WB, Bloomston M, et al. Long-term efficacy of lymph node reoperation for persistent papillary thyroid cancer. J Clin Endocrinol Metab. 2010;95:2187–94.
35. Mazzaferri EL, Young RL, Oertel JE, et al. Papillary thyroid carcinoma: the impact of therapy in 576 patients. Medicine (Baltimore). 1977;56:171–96.
36. Robenshtok E, Fish S, Bach A, et al. Suspicious cervical lymph nodes detected after thyroidectomy for papillary thyroid cancer usually remain stable over years in properly selected patients. J Clin Endocrinol Metab. 2012;97:2706–13.
37. Rondeau G, Fish S, Hann LE, et al. Ultrasonographically detected small thyroid bed nodules identified after total thyroidectomy for differentiated thyroid cancer seldom show clinically significant structural progression. Thyroid. 2011;21:845–53.
38. Nixon IJ, Ganly I, Patel S, et al. The impact of microscopic extrathyroid extension on outcome in patients with clinical T1 and T2 well-differentiated thyroid cancer. Surgery. 2011;150:1242–9.
39. Sawka AM, Straus S, Gafni A, et al. How can we meet the information needs of patients with early stage papillary thyroid cancer considering radioactive iodine remnant ablation? Clin Endocrinol. 2011;74:419–23.
40. Sawka AM, Straus S, Rotstein L, et al. Randomized controlled trial of a computerized decision aid on adjuvant radioactive iodine treatment for patients with early-stage papillary thyroid cancer. J Clin Oncol. 2012;30:2906–11.
41. Carty SE, Doherty GM, Inabnet III WB, et al. American Thyroid Association statement on the essential elements of interdisciplinary communication of perioperative information for patients undergoing thyroid cancer surgery. Thyroid. 2012;22:395–9.
42. Weinrib SL, Lane WS, Rappaport JM. Successful management of differentiated thyroid cancer in a community-based endocrine practice. Endocr Pract. 2012;18:170–8.
43. Xing M. BRAF mutation in thyroid cancer. Endocr Relat Cancer. 2005;12:245–62.
44. Romei C, Elisei R. RET/PTC translocations and clinico-pathological features in human papillary thyroid carcinoma. Front Endocrinol (Lausanne). 2012;3:54.

45. Alexander EK, Kennedy GC, Baloch ZW, et al. Preoperative diagnosis of benign thyroid nodules with indeterminate cytology. N Engl J Med. 2012;367:705–15.
46. Schlumberger M. Target therapies for radioiodine refractory advanced thyroid tumors. J Endocrinol Invest. 2012;35(6 Suppl):40–4.
47. Berwick DM. The science of improvement. JAMA. 2008;299:1182–4.
48. Livingston EH, McNutt RA. The hazards of evidence-based medicine assessing variations in care. JAMA. 2011;306:762–3.

Medullary Thyroid Cancer

8

Laura Chin-Lenn and Janice L. Pasieka

Introduction

Medullary thyroid cancer (MTC) is an uncommon disease, accounting for 3–10 % of all thyroid cancers worldwide [1–3]. The German literature contains reports of a thyroid malignancy with amyloid deposits as early as 1906, but it was not until 1959 when Hazard and co-workers reported on a clinicopathological, solid arrangement of cells, which represented medullary (solid) carcinoma [4, 5]. Seventy per cent of MTCs are sporadic, whereas 30 % have a germline mutation of the RET proto-oncogene, which leads to various familial forms of this disease.

Pathology

MTC arises from neural crest-derived C-cells (previously known as parafollicular cells) of the thyroid gland. As a result of shared embryological derivation, MTC secretes neuroendocrine peptides and shares a few similar clinical and histological characteristics with other neuroendocrine cells. It is now thought that C-cells might be differentiated from an endodermal component that also derives from other neuroendocrine cells of the respiratory and gastrointestinal tract [6]. C-cells account for <0.1 % of thyroid epithelial weight and occur adjacent to follicles throughout the gland, with a higher concentration in the middle-third of the lateral lobes and with a paucity of cells in the isthmus [7]. Calcitonin from the C-cells is stimulated by increased calcium and mainly acts to suppress calcium release by inhibiting bone resorption.

L. Chin-Lenn (✉) • J.L. Pasieka
Section of General Surgery and Surgical Oncology, University of Calgary,
1403 29 St NW, Calgary, AB T2N 2 T9, Canada
e-mail: lchinlenn@hotmail.com; Janice.pasieka@albertahealthservices.ca

© K. Alok Pathak, Richard W. Nason, Janice L. Pasieka, Rehan Kazi,
Raghav C. Dwivedi 2015
Springer India/Byword Books
K.A. Pathak et al. (eds.), *Management of Thyroid Cancer: Special Considerations*,
Head and Neck Cancer Clinics, DOI 10.1007/978-81-322-2434-1_8

Fig. 8.1 Calcitonin stain
showing C-cell hyperplasia
(Courtesy of Dr Moosa
Khalil)

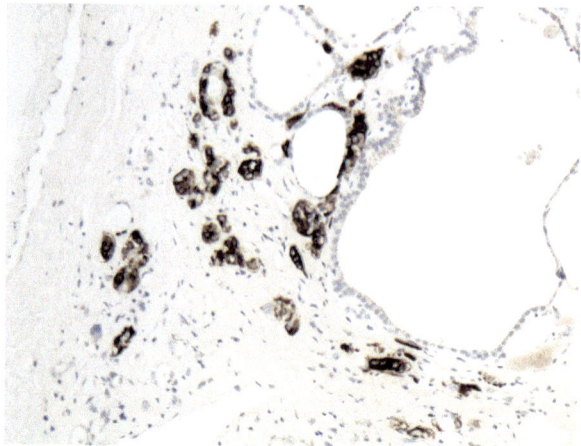

Fig. 8.2 Resected thyroid
showing medullary thyroid
cancer in the left lobe
(Courtesy of Dr Moosa
Khalil)

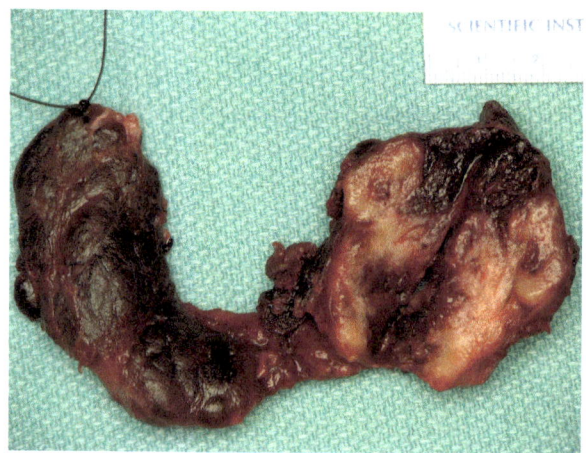

C-cell hyperplasia (CCH) was described initially as occurring in 'knots and clusters' with each cell being hypertrophic. Although it varies throughout the literature, the modern pathological definition is of C-cell hyperplasia is >6 C-cells per follicle or >50 C-cells per low power field (Fig. 8.1) [8]. C-cell hyperplasia can be found in up to a third of 'normal' thyroids or unrelated to MTC (such as in chronic lymphocytic thyroiditis, neonatal or elderly patients, or hyperparathyroidism); however, in the familial setting of MTC it is considered a premalignant condition akin to carcinoma in situ [6, 9, 10].

MTCs are most frequently located posteriorly at the junction between the upper-third and lower two-thirds of the lateral lobes of the thyroid where the C-cells are concentrated. They are usually firm, white or grey, and well defined but unencapsulated (Fig. 8.2). Cells can be variable in shape and mildly pleomorphic but nuclei are characteristic of other neuroendocrine tumours, with round-oval shape with a fine stippled 'salt and pepper' nuclear chromatin (Fig. 8.3a). Calcification and

Fig. 8.3 (**a**) Haematoxylin and eosin stain of medullary thyroid cancer. (**b**) Congo red stain under polarized light showing amyloid in medullary thyroid cancer (Courtesy of Dr Moosa Khalil)

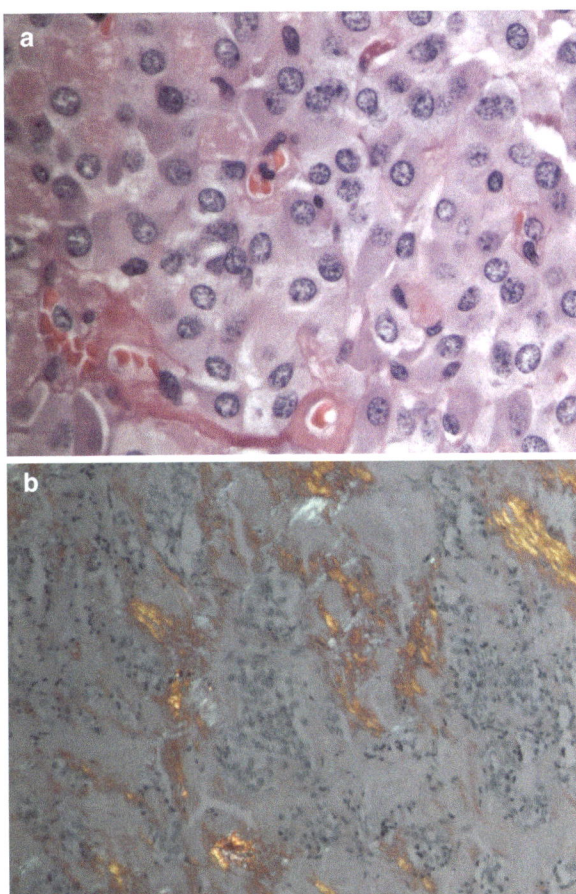

surrounding amyloid (composed of full-length calcitonin) might be present (Fig. 8.3b) [11, 12].

Genetic Testing

The 21 exon RET proto-oncogene on chromosome 10q11.2 was first described in 1985 [13]. The RET proto-oncogene encodes the RET (rearranged during transfection) protein, a receptor tyrosine kinase (RTK) that is expressed in neural crest-origin derivatives [14]. There are 17–20 classes of 58 RTKs that also include vascular endothelial growth factor (VEGF) and endothelial-derived growth factor receptor (EGFR). RTKs consist of a ligand-binding extracellular portion, a cysteine-rich region necessary for receptor dimerization, a transmembrane domain, and an intracellular portion consisting of two tyrosine kinase (TK) regions that activate intracellular signal transduction pathways (Fig. 8.4) [15]. Activation triggers

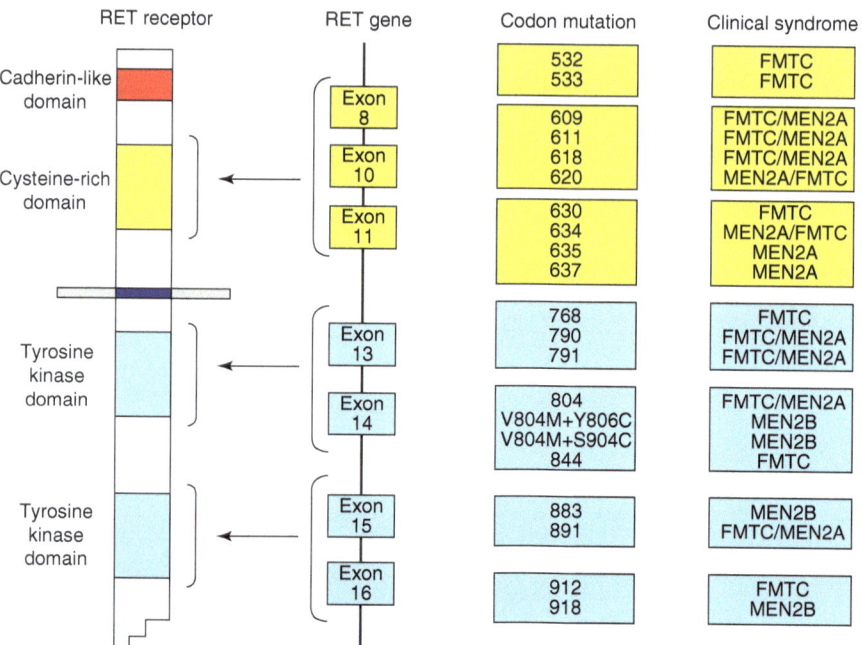

Fig. 8.4 Diagram of the RET receptor, gene and corresponding codon mutations and their associ-ated clinical syndromes (Reproduced with permission from Hubner and Houlston [15])

autophosphorylation of the extracellular tyrosine residues that serve as docking sites for adaptor proteins, which coordinate intracellular signal transduction path-ways that are important in regulating cell growth [1–3, 14].

Germline point mutations in the RET proto-oncogene can be identified in 95 % of cases of MEN2 (multiple endocrine neoplasia type 2), which suggests that undis-covered additional loci may exist (Fig. 8.4). In sporadic MTC, germline RET muta-tions are uncommon (1.5–24 %) but somatic RET mutations occur in 25–50 % of cases [4, 5, 16–18].

Hereditary MTC

Hereditary forms of MTC account for ~30 % of MTC. MEN2A and 2B are inherited in an autosomal dominant fashion with complete penetrance for MTC. MTC can present at any age but is most common in the second to fourth decades [6, 19]. It is usually the first presentation of the syndrome and is often multicentric and bilateral. Genetic testing may also reveal family members positive for germline mutations who can be considered for prophylactic surgery before the development of MTC.

MEN2A (Sipple syndrome) is the most common variant of MEN2, occurring in 80–90 % of familial MTC. The most common codon mutation is 634 (80 %). The

MEN2A consists of MTC (>90 %), pheochromocytoma (50 %) and primary hyper-parathyroidism (15–30 %). Index cases of MTC often present with a thyroid or neck mass between the ages of 15 and 20 years, although it has been observed in children as young as 5 years of age [7, 20]. Variations of MEN2A also occur uncommonly with RET codon 634 mutation with cutaneous lichen amyloidosis (upper back cuta-neous pruritic lesion) or with Hirschprung disease [8, 21, 22].

Familial MTC (FMTC) was described initially in 1986 in two families who were developed a more indolent form of MTC at a later age (~43 years old) with no other clinical manifestations of the MEN2 syndrome [6, 9, 10, 23]. The penetrance of MTC is lower than that of MEN2A and occurs at an older age. Definition of FMTC varies from greater than four members in family with MTC without pheochromocy-toma or hyperparathyroidism to more stringent guidelines of more than 10 carriers with multiple carriers, or affected members over the age of 50 years [11, 12, 19, 24]. The stricter criteria aim to avoid mislabelling late occurring MEN2A as FMTC and potentially miss a pheochromocytoma [13, 19]. This may also account for the dif-ference in the incidence of FMTC and MEN2A in the literature. In a large series, 75 % of FMTC presented as apparently sporadic cases [14, 25]. For this reason, FMTC could be considered as a variant of MEN2A with decreased penetrance for pheochromocytoma and hyperparathyroidism, rather than as its own entity.

MEN2B occurs in 5–20 % of MEN2 patients. Features include: (i) MTC; (ii) pheochromocytoma; (iii) marfanoid habitus (without Marfan syndrome); (iv) pes cavus; (v) pectus excavatum; (vi) hypotonia; (vii) proximal muscle weakness; (viii) mucosal neuromas on the lips, anterolateral surface of tongue and conjunctiva; (ix) medullated corneal nerves; and (x) intestinal ganglioneuromatosis [24]. The most common mutation is codon 918 in 95 % of patients with MEN2B. Approximately 50 % of MEN2B patients have de novo germline RET mutations, usually of paternal origin [26]. In MEN2B, both MTC and pheochromocytoma are more aggressive variants that occur at an earlier age compared with MEN2A.

Pheochromocytoma in MEN2 are usually bilateral (≤78 %), rarely metastasize (<5 %), and half are asymptomatic. Annual surveillance with 24-h urine metaneph-rines or plasma-free metanephrines is recommended from the age of 8 years for MEN2B and codons 630 and 634, and by the age of 20 years for other MEN2A mutations. The difficulty with surveillance lies in differentiating pheochromocy-toma from its precursor—adrenal medullary hyperplasia—when a patient has ele-vated biochemical tests but an absence of localizing imaging [20].

Before the era of genetic testing, screening those at high-risk for familial MTC was with yearly calcitonin and pentagastrin-stimulated calcitonin levels, 24-h uri-nary metanephrines, serum calcium, and parathyroid hormone (PTH) measurement in 6–35-year-olds. Currently, all first-degree relatives of known germline RET mutation carriers should be offered genetic testing before the age of recommended prophylactic surgery [27]. DNA is specifically examined for the exons commonly involved with MEN2, eliminating the need for yearly screening of all family mem-bers. The guidelines recommend that children who are positive for RET mutation undergo prophylactic thyroidectomy. Many ethical considerations surround genetic testing and prophylactic surgery at such a young age, but the accuracy of RET

Table 8.1 Prophylactic surgery by codon mutation

ATA risk level	Codons	Subtype	RET testing	Age for ultrasound	Age for first serum calcitonin	Age for surgery
D (highest risk)	883 918	MEN2B	ASAP, within 1st year of life	ASAP, within 1st year of life	6 months if surgery not already performed	ASAP, within 1st year of life
C	634	MEN2A	<3–5 years	>3–5 years	>3–5 years	Before 5 years lymph node dissection controversial
B	609 611 618 620 630	MEN2A FMTC	<3–5 years	>3–5 years	>3–5 years	Total thyroidectomy 5–10 years; some suggest by 5 years
A (lower risk)	768 790 790 804 891	MEN2A FMTC	<3–5 years	>3–5 years	>3–5 years	Total thyroidectomy 5–10 years

Note: Adapted from the American Thyroid Association guidelines [27]

testing is high (95 % for MEN2 and 88 % for FMTC), penetrance of MTC is 100 %, and surgery is the only chance for cure [28]. The location of the RET codon mutation can predict biological behaviour, and guidelines stratifying codon types into four risk levels have been established to direct the timing of prophylactic surgery (Table 8.1).

Prophylactic surgery for paediatric MEN2 patients (ATA-A – D) with no evidence of metastases is total thyroidectomy. MEN2B patients treated after the age of 1 year should also undergo a prophylactic central compartment dissection. Preoperatively, elevated serum calcitonin of >40 pg/ml or MTC size of ≥5 mm indicate the need for investigation for distant metastases, although the accuracy of calcitonin to predict metastases in very young patients is unknown. Therapeutic dissection of positive lymph node compartments should be undertaken.

Primary hyperparathyroidism in MEN2A can be solitary or multiple and is more likely to coexist if codon 634 mutation is present. Normal parathyroid glands should be tagged and left in situ, if possible. In MEN2A, abnormal parathyroid glands seen at MTC surgery should be treated with a parathyroidectomy and autograft into the forearm, as if the patient has mild hyperparathyroidism, even if the patient is normocalcaemic [19]. This will also protect the parathyroid function in the event of reoperative surgery for either recurrent MTC or hyperparathyroidism. For MEN2B or FMTC, devascularized parathyroids should be autotransplanted. Some surgeons leave the parathyroid glands in situ when treating hereditary MTCs if the patient is <8 years old, as they have found the risk of nodal metastases to be is low [29].

Newly Detected Cases of MTC

MTC may be detected during routine screening when calcitonin is used to monitor thyroid nodular disease, a practice that has caused much debate. Large European series have found a 0.4–0.6 % incidence of elevated calcitonin in thyroid nodules with fine-needle aspiration (FNA) that is not diagnostic of MTC [30, 31]. These patients were appropriately treated for MTC at an earlier stage with subsequent postoperative calcitonin normalization [30, 31]. However, screening calcitonin, especially when only mildly elevated, might lead to surgery for CCH or even benign disease [32]. Although calcitonin has good sensitivity for diagnosing MTC, confirmation with a pentagastrin stimulation test has been suggested [33]. In North America where pentagastrin is unavailable, interpretation of mildly elevated calcitonin levels is difficult [34]. Calcium-stimulated calcitonin has been shown in relatively smaller studies to be well tolerated, and stimulated-calcitonin levels distinguishing normal, CCH and MTC have been identified [35]. Screening for calcitonin appears to be cost-effective in evaluation models in both Europe and USA [36, 37]. Despite the earlier recommendation for screening calcitonin, the most recent European guidelines are less enthusiastic and instead suggest that it might be a useful nodular disease while the National Comprehensive Cancer Network (NCCN) guidelines have remained equivocal [27, 38].

Sporadic MTC accounts for 70 % of MTCs and usually presents in the fifth/sixth decade of life as a palpable thyroid mass or lymph node (LN), anterior neck pain, compressive symptoms of hoarseness, dysphagia or dyspnoea or hormonal symptoms, such as flushing or diarrhoea. [39] A thorough history should be taken with emphasis on the possibility of previously undetected familial disease. At presentation, LN involvement occurs in 35–50 % of patients and distant metastases in 10–15 %, most commonly in the lungs, mediastinum, liver, bone and less commonly to brain and skin.

Investigations to assess locoregional disease include high-resolution ultrasound of the thyroid, central and bilateral lateral LN compartments, and superior mediastinum. FNA of suspicious nodules or LNs should be undertaken. The accuracy of FNA for MTC is lower than that in differentiated thyroid cancer, with only 62 % sensitivity [40]. As an adjunct, following the FNA, the needle can be washed in 1 ml of normal saline and sent for calcitonin testing (calcitonin washout). This can detect MTC in thyroid nodules and metastatic LNs with almost 100 % sensitivity and specificity [40].

Serum tumour markers, in particular calcitonin, aid in staging, follow-up and prognosis. Calcitonin levels correlate with tumour burden, LN metastases (likely if calcitonin levels between 10–40 pg/ml), and distant metastases (highly likely if >1,000 pg/ml) [41, 42]. Preoperative serum carcino-embryonic antigen (CEA) might also correlate with tumour burden [43]. Serum chromogranin A, often used to detect neuroendocrine tumours, has limited utility in MTC, as it is elevated only in advanced disease [44].

All patients with MTC, CCH or MEN2 should be offered genetic testing for germline RET mutations of known MEN2-related exons. New patients presenting with apparently sporadic MTC have germline RET mutations in 4–6.5 % and 41.1 % of their tested relatives are gene carriers [45, 46]. Routine testing for somatic RET mutations is not currently recommended by the NCCN guidelines, although their presence may indicate a more advanced stage at diagnosis with worse prognosis for persistent disease and death, although this has not been correlated in all studies [45].

Preoperatively, pheochromocytoma should be excluded with either negative RET testing, 24-h urinary metanephrines, or plasma meta-nephrines and adrenal imaging with CT or MRI. If pheochromocytoma is diagnosed, it must be treated with appropriate preoperative alpha-blockade before MTC to avoid the complication of an intraoperative adrenergic crisis. Serum calcium and PTH should be measured before surgery to exclude primary hyperparathyroidism and aid in surgical planning.

Management of Locoregional Disease

Surgery for disease confined to the thyroid (T1-3, N0, M0) is total thyroidectomy and prophylactic central (level VI) LN dissection. In unilateral palpable MTC, central LNs are involved in 81 % [47]. The central compartment has been defined as the carotid sheaths laterally, the hyoid superiorly, the innominate artery or sternal notch inferiorly, and the superficial and deep layers of the deep cervical fascia anteriorly and posteriorly [48].

Lateral neck dissection (therapeutic) is recommended if there is suspicion of lateral LN disease either clinically or radiologically in those LN basins. For those with palpable LN at presentation, the rate of LN involvement has been found to be high, with 100 % central compartment, 93 % ipsilateral lateral, 45 % contralateral, and 52 % mediastinal involvement [49]. The importance of preoperative high-resolution ultrasound is emphasized, as it is difficult even for experienced surgeons to reliably identify LN metastases intraoperatively by palpation and inspection (sensitivity 64 %, specificity 71 %) [47].

The role of prophylactic lateral LN dissection is controversial. The recent ATA guidelines have recognized, with value of ultrasound to predict disease in the lateral compartments and suggest FNA of suspicious nodes and subsequent compartment dissection, only for proven positive disease [27]. However, proponents of prophylactic lateral LN dissection argue that in the absence of effective adjuvant therapy for a disease with high rates of occult LN metastases, surgery should be thorough. In unilobar MTC, ipsilateral lateral LN metastases occur in 57–81 % and contralateral disease in 28–44 % [47, 50] The risk of LN metastases in multifocal disease is at least doubled compared with unifocal disease [51]. Although the size of MTC has been found to be a predictor of LN involvement, it is inconsistent [50, 52].

Involved central compartment LNs may predict the presence and number of ipsilateral and to a lesser extent contralateral lateral LN metastases [53]. Contralateral LNs are usually only involved in addition to positive central and ipsilateral lateral LNs [53]. LN status may also be able to predict an undetectable postoperative calcitonin with 95 % undetectable without LN metastases, and 32 % with LN metastases [50]. Bilateral lateral LN dissection may be considered in the presence of extensive ipsilateral lateral LN disease [54]. However, despite extensive surgery with its concomitant risks, even N0 patients may not have calcitonin normalized in 38 % of them, which makes the benefit of prophylactic lateral LN dissection questionable [42]. An alternative strategy might be to initially defer the prophylactic lateral LN dissection until postoperative calcitonin levels are indicative of surgery.

Mediastinal metastatic LN may indicate systemic disease and confer poor prognosis; thus suspicious upper mediastinal nodes should be removed via the cervical incision, if possible [55, 56]. Compartment-orientated dissection of mediastinal LN via a trans-sternal approach has been performed previously by some groups, but is now considered only in exceptional circumstances [56].

In the presence of extensive local disease or distant metastases, surgery might be less aggressive and tailored to a more palliative approach aiming to minimize complications and to control symptoms, such as pain or airway compromise. Diagnostic laparoscopy has been used to detect liver metastases that are too small to be seen on cross-sectional imaging [57]. Surgery should be planned by bearing in mind staging and predicted survival with their burden of metastatic disease. Systemic therapies or clinical trials may be considered.

Staging and Prognosis

Staging is important to plan the extent of surgery, as a less aggressive approach may be taken in the setting of locally advanced or advanced metastatic disease. Investigations for distant metastases are CT of the neck and mediastinum with additional CT of the abdomen and pelvis if calcitonin is >400 pg/ml. The AJCC TNM staging is listed in Tables 8.2 and 8.3.

Overall, 5-year disease-specific survival ranges from 83 to 86 % and 10-year survival from 72 to 78 % [59–61]. The only consistent predictors of survival on multivariate analysis are stage of disease and age at diagnosis [60, 62].

Incidentally Detected MTC

Around 10–15 % of MTC are found incidentally after a thyroidectomy for other indications, such as multinodular goitre (0.3 %), FNA that reveals indeterminate nodules (1–2 %), or concurrently with a differentiated cancer [63]. A systematic review of 24 autopsy series revealed occult MTC in 0.14 % of autopsies [64].

Patients already treated with hemithyroidectomy should be subject to the same preoperative investigations as clinically detected MTC. Particular attention should be paid to the pathology, especially concomitant CCH, multifocal disease, extrathyroidal extension and margin status. In the presence of elevated calcitonin or positive RET germline mutation, completion thyroidectomy with central and, if indicated, lateral LN dissection should be performed. If the patient has negative surgical margins, undetectable serum calcitonin, no evidence of persistent disease in the neck, or

Table 8.2 American Joint Committee on Cancer—tumour, node, metastasis (TNM) staging for thyroid cancer [58]

Primary tumour (T)	
Tx	Primary tumour cannot be assessed
T0	No evidence of primary tumour
T1	Tumour ≤2 cm in greatest dimension, limited to the thyroid
T1a	Tumour ≤1 cm, limited to the thyroid
T1b	Tumour >1 cm but not >2 cm in greatest dimension, limited to the thyroid
T2	Tumour >2 cm but not >4 cm in greatest dimension, limited to the thyroid
T3	Tumour >4 cm in greatest dimension, limited to the thyroid or any tumour with minimal extrathyroid extension (e.g., extension to sternothyroid muscle or perithyroid soft tissues)
T4a	Moderately advanced disease
	Tumour of any size extending beyond the thyroid capsule to invade subcutaneous soft tissues, larynx, trachea, oesophagus, or recurrent laryngeal nerve
T4b	Very advanced disease
	Tumour invades prevertebral fascia or encases the carotid artery or mediastinal vessels
Regional lymph nodes (N)	
Nx	Regional lymph nodes cannot be assessed
N0	No regional lymph node metastasis
N1	Regional lymph node metastasis
N1a	Metastasis to level VI (pretracheal, paratracheal and prelaryngeal/Delphian lymph nodes)
N1b	Metastasis to unilateral, bilateral or contralateral cervical (levels I, II, III, IV or V) or retropharyngeal or superior mediastinal lymph nodes (level VII)
Distant metastasis (M)	
M0	No distant metastasis
M1	Distant metastasis

Reproduced with permission from Edge et al. [58] 89

CCH, and is therefore judged to be at low-risk for residual disease, either surgery or clinical follow-up are reasonable approaches.

Follow-Up

Postoperatively, patients should have thyroxine replacement in the therapeutic range. Two to 3 months following surgery, clinical examination should be undertaken and postoperative serum calcitonin and CEA measured. Postoperative stimulated calcitonin is no longer widely used. The half-life of serum calcitonin is short, probably ~10 min, but levels may take time to fall with postulated reasons being slow release from thyroidal and extrathyroidal storage, or possible interference of some calcitonin assays with calcitonin precursors [65]. It is thus recommended to measure the postoperative calcitonin 2–3 months after surgery [27]. Calcitonin normalization (biochemical cure) occurs in 43–49 % of patients and may be predicted

Table 8.3 American Joint Committee on Cancer Stage Grouping [58] and Survival for Medullary Thyroid Carcinoma [1, 59, 60]

Stage group	T stage	N stage	M stage	5-year survival (%)
Stage I	T1	N0	M0	98–100
Stage II	T2	N0	M0	93–100
Stage III	T3	N0	M0	66–73
	T1	N1a	M0	
	T2	N1a	M0	
	T3	N1a	M0	
Stage IV				21–48
Stage IVA	TIa	N0	M0	
	TIa	N1a	M0	
	T1	N1b	M0	
	T2	N1b	M0	
	T3	N1b	M0	
	T4a	N1b	M0	
Stage IVB	T4b	Any N	M0	
Stage IVC	Any T	Any N	M1	

Reproduced with permission from Edge et al. [58]:89

by stage at surgery [54, 59, 60], preoperative calcitonin [66] and the number of positive LN [67]. In patients without LN metastases, serum calcitonin is undetectable in 60–90 % compared with <20 % in the presence of LN metastases [42]. Survival of patients who have biochemical cure is better than those who have persistently elevated calcitonin, with 10-year clinical remission of 90 % [68] and survival of 97.7 % vs. 70 % [59]. Of those who achieve biochemical cure, 3.3–12 % will have a biochemical recurrence with subsequent elevation of calcitonin [54, 59, 69]. If calcitonin is undetectable, routine follow-up should consist of 6 month to yearly physical examination with neck ultrasound and serum calcitonin and CEA, with imaging reserved for those with detected abnormalities.

Calcitonin doubling times correlate with prognosis, predicting recurrence, tumour progression and overall survival [42, 70–72]. A meta-analysis found that both calcitonin and CEA are strong negative predictors of recurrence-free and disease-related survival, particularly for doubling times of <1 year [73]. CEA may be a marker of dedifferentiation if it continues to rise despite a low calcitonin doubling time [74].

A major challenge in the management of MTC is persistent disease with elevated calcitonin in spite of seemingly adequate surgery, which occurs in ≤50 % of patients [29, 68, 75]. If the calcitonin is elevated a thorough review of the operative note, physical examination and high resolution neck ultrasound should be undertaken.

The rate of detection increases with increasing CEA and calcitonin, and conversely is more likely to be inconclusive with lower levels [42, 76]. If calcitonin is >150 pg/ml, re-imaging for distant metastases—particularly lung, mediastinum, liver and bone—should be performed with CT of the neck, chest and abdomen, dedicated triple-phase CT or MRI of the liver, bone MRI of the spine and pelvis, and bone scan. Bone scan may be better in peripheral bony metastases [76]. The role of 18F-FDG PET scanning is unclear. It has been shown that sensitivity is higher (78 %) with calcitonin levels of >1,000 pg/ml while its use is limited if calcitonin levels are <500 pg/ml [77]. In a series comparing CT, MRI and PET, PET was found overall to be less accurate, particularly for lung and liver and bone metastases [76]. PET/CT using other isotopes, in particular 18-F DOPA, have been investigated and found to be superior to 18F-FDG at detecting metastases overall (18F-DOPA 85–94 % vs. 18F-FDG 28–62 %) and in liver and bone [78, 79]. Previous studies showed that 18F-FDG may be better for patients with rapid calcium doubling time (<24 months) [80]. The use of 68Ga-DOTA-NOC PET-CT has not shown any significant benefits over 18F-FDG PET/CT [81, 82]. Recently, it has been reported that [111]Inoctreotide scintigraphy for metastatic MTC in the paediatric population is less sensitive than conventional imaging [83].

Tisell et al. initially described reoperative cervical surgery for 11 patients with persistently elevated postoperative calcitonin, consisting of meticulous microdissection of the central and lateral neck compartment to thoroughly remove all tissue, including microscopic MTC metastases, with 4 patients having normalized calcitonin levels [84]. Reoperative surgery is technically challenging with inherent risks. In a large series of 147 patients with hypoparathyroidism (3 %), injury to the recurrent laryngeal nerve was reported in 2 % and thoracic duct injury in 5 % of patients [75]. Temporary paresis of the axillary nerve, hypoglossal nerve and sympathetic trunk (Horner syndrome) can also occur [85].

Reoperative surgery is often unrewarding, with early reports of poor rates of biochemical cure and high rates of recurrent disease, which led some to authors to suggest a conservative route of management [86]. However, Moley et al. showed that by improving staging, particularly with diagnostic laparoscopy, patients with only local or regional disease could be selected for surgery with improvement in calcitonin normalization from 28 to 38 %, and reduction of the rate of calcitonin non-response from 31 to 13 % [87]. Long-term follow-up by the same group showed durable rates of decreased calcitonin of <10 pg/ml (26 %) over 8–10 years, with an additional 20 % with calcitonin of <100 pg/ml with no evidence of recurrence in either group [75].

Despite detectable serum calcitonin postoperatively, long-term survival can be good if levels remain stable (at 5 years 90 % and 10 years 85 %) [86].

Treatment for Distant Metastases

The best chance for cure of MTC is with primary surgery. Outcomes of adjuvant treatment for metastatic disease have generally been discouraging. Although external beam radiotherapy (EBRT) does not improve overall survival, it may decrease local recurrence when used as adjuvant therapy with adequate surgery for patients in high-risk populations (residual microscopic disease, extraglandular invasion, LN involvement) [88–92]. Palliative EBRT can also be used for inoperable local disease, gross incomplete resection of locally advanced disease, and palliation of bony metastases.

Studies in chemotherapy for MTC have been few with results being mostly limited to disease stabilization and partial response of relatively short duration. Targeted therapies are now being considered as the initial choice, if possible, for metastatic MTC, with recent phase III trials showing promising results. Tyrosine kinase (TK) inhibitors are small organic compounds that can be specific to one or several TK receptors. They affect the TK-dependent oncogenic pathways by competing with the adenosine triphosphate (ATP) binding site of the catalytic domain of TK, which inhibits phosphorylation and activation of TK and prevents further activation of intracellular signalling pathways.

A recent phase III trial for metastatic MTC administered vandetanib to 231 people with MTC and 100 placebo with open-label crossover for progression in the placebo group. Treatment improved median progressionfree survival (19.3 months placebo vs. 30.5 months vandetanib) with advantages in objective response (45 % vs. 13 %), disease control rate (87 % vs. 71 %), and biochemical response (calcitonin 69 vs. 3 % and CEA 52 vs.2 %) [93]. Targeted therapies are further discussed in Chapter 11.

CEA has been used with some promise as a target for pretargeted radioimmunotherapy in patients with progressing metastatic MTC. A bispecific monoclonal antibody (CEA-labelled) is administered, followed a few days later by a radiolabelled bivalent hapten (often ^{131}I-labelled) that binds to the cells targeted by the initial antibody. A comparison of 29 patients with contemporaneous controls found that in high-risk patients (with calcitonin doubling times <2 years) the overall survival was significantly higher (metastatic MTC group 110 months vs. controls 61 months) [94]. A phase II trial of 42 patients with progressive metastatic MTC showed disease control rates (objective response and stable disease) of 76.2 %, with 21/37 patients having prolongation of CEA and calcitonin doubling time with subsequent benefits in survival [95].

The fact that some neuroendocrine tumours, including MTC, show uptake on mIBG or somatostatin receptor scintigraphy, radionucleide therapy has been investigated, particularly with DOTA-TOC and mIBG. DOTA-TOC labelled to ^{90}Y was administered to 21 patients and had 29 % response rate, with those patients showing improved survival (75 vs. 11 months from time of therapy) [96]. MIBG for diagnostic use is limited, having only 30 % sensitivity, although >90 % specificity. Therapeutically, it can be used to slow disease progression. In a series of 13 patients with metastatic MTC in whom mIBG uptake was demonstrated, 4 patients had a partial response and 4 had stable disease [97]. The other role of radionuclide therapy is for symptom palliation of patients with progressive metastatic neuroendocrine tumours [98].

The treatment of metastatic disease is discussed in detail in a separate chapter. Symptom control for these patients is important as the course of metastatic disease may be prolonged. Diarrhoea can be controlled with loperamide, codeine or somatostatin analogues [99]. Pain needs to be controlled with analgesia but palliative surgery may be indicated for painful or compressive metastases or hormonal secretion. Symptom relief from widely metastatic disease may be achieved with cytoreductive surgery [100]. Bony metastases may be palliated with surgery, EBRT, mIBG or possibly bisphosphonates. Treatment of liver metastases includes laparoscopic radiofrequency ablation (RFA) and transarterial chemoembolization with epirubicin [101–103].

Summary

MTC is an uncommon disease, which can occur from hereditary and sporadic factors. If present, germline mutations may predict the clinical course and indicate the timing for prophylactic surgery. Tumour markers, in particular calcitonin and CEA, are useful for diagnosis, follow-up and prognosis. At present, surgery is the only effective treatment for curative intent. Although adjuvant therapy has historically had poor results, promising developments, in particular with targeted therapy, are on the horizon.

Commentary

Richard W. Nason

The diagnosis of medullary thyroid cancer (MTC) has several important implications. The extent of disease in the neck needs to be evaluated, preferably with a combination of ultrasound and CT scan. Screening for pheochromocytoma and hyperparathyroidism needs to be done and the RET proto-oncogene should be analysed to determine whether the disease is sporadic or hereditary.

The primary treatment of MTC is surgical removal of all neoplastic tissue in the neck after exclusion of a pheochromocytoma. Maximizing local and regional control is important. Total thyroidectomy is generally accepted for the hereditary and sporadic forms of the disease. Elective central compartment neck dissection is also accepted. Elective treatment of the lateral neck is controversial. The authors prophylactically dissect the lateral neck in the presence of clinically positive central compartment nodes. MTC is associated with relatively long survival, irrespective of the extent of elective treatment of the neck at the time of presentation. A unique feature of this disease is the sensitive tumour markers, calcitonin and CEA, for persistent and recurrent disease. They are, in fact, so sensitive that they can complicate management. A rise in these markers posttreatment in an otherwise asymptomatic patient creates a dilemma and serves to emphasize the importance of adequate initial surgery. The approach to the rising tumour markers is again controversial: How much and what investigations? Is reoperation on the neck necessary? In the authors' opinion imaging of the neck with reoperation for clinically evident disease is appropriate. An extensive search for asymptomatic distant metastases has to be tempered with the knowledge that distant metastases have no curative treatment. If reoperation on the neck is contemplated for minimal neck disease, then exclusion of distant disease is acceptable. It is important to emphasize that long-term survival is good in the presence of stable tumour markers.

References

1. Hundahl SA, Fleming ID, Fremgen AM, et al. A national cancer database report on 53,856 cases of thyroid carcinoma treated in the US, 1985–1995. Cancer. 1998;83:2638–48.
2. Saad MF, Ordonez NG, Rashid RK, et al. Medullary carcinoma of the thyroid. A study of the clinical features and prognostic factors in 161 patients. Medicine (Baltimore). 1984;63:319–42.
3. Aschebrook-Kilfoy B, Ward MH, Sabra MM, et al. Thyroid cancer incidence patterns in the United States by histologic type, 1992–2006. Thyroid. 2011;21:125–34.
4. Hazard JB. The C-cells (parafollicular cells) of the thyroid gland and medullary thyroid carcinoma: a review. Am J Pathol. 1977;88:213–50.
5. Hazard JB, Hawk WA, Crile G. Medullary (solid) carcinoma of the thyroid: a clinicopathologic entity. J Clin Endocrinol Metab. 1959;19:152–61.
6. Albores-Saavedra JA, Krueger JE. C-cell hyperplasia and medullary thyroid microcarcinoma. Endocr Pathol. 2001;12:365–77.
7. Wolfe HJ, Voelkel EF, Tashjian AH. Distribution of calcitonin-containing cells in the normal adult human thyroid gland: a correlation of morphology with peptide content. J Clin Endocrinol Metab. 1974;38:688–94.
8. Chen H, Sippel RS, O'Dorisio MS, et al. The North American Neuroendocrine Tumor Society consensus guideline for the diagnosis and management of neuroendocrine tumors: pheochromocytoma, paraganglioma, and medullary thyroid cancer. Pancreas. 2010;39:775–83.
9. Machens A, Niccoli-Sire P, Hoegel J, et al. Early malignant progression of hereditary medullary thyroid cancer. N Engl J Med. 2003;349:1517–25.
10. Guyétant S, Dupre F, Bigorgne JC, et al. Medullary thyroid microcarcinoma: a clinicopathologic retrospective study of 38 patients with no prior familial disease. Hum Pathol. 1999;30:957–63.
11. Thompson LDR. Medullary thyroid carcinoma. Ear Nose Throat J. 2010;89:301–2.
12. Khurana R. Unraveling the amyloid associated with human medullary thyroid carcinoma. Endocrinology. 2004;145:5465–70.
13. Takahashi M, Ritz J, Cooper GM. Activation of a novel human transforming gene, ret, by DNA rearrangement. Cell. 1985;42:581–8.
14. Eng C. RET proto-oncogene in the development of human cancer. J Clin Oncol. 1999;17:380–93.
15. Hubner RA, Houlston RS. Molecular advances in medullary thyroid cancer diagnostics. Clin Chim Acta. 2006;370:2–8.
16. Eng C, Mulligan LM, Smith DP, et al. Low frequency of germline mutations in the RET proto-oncogene in patients with apparently sporadic medullary thyroid carcinoma. Clin Endocrinol. 1995;43:123–7.
17. Elisei R, Cosci B, Romei C, et al. Prognostic significance of somatic RET oncogene mutations in sporadic medullary thyroid cancer: a 10-year follow-up study. J Clin Endocrinol Metab. 2007;93:682–7.
18. Marsh DJ, Learoyd DL, Andrew SD, et al. Somatic mutations in the RET protooncogene in sporadic medullary thyroid carcinoma. Clin Endocrinol. 1996;44:249–57.
19. Brandi ML, Gagel RF, Angeli A, et al. Guidelines for diagnosis and therapy of MEN type 1 and type 2. J Clin Endocrinol Metab. 2001;86:5658–71.
20. Kouvaraki MA, Shapiro SE, Perrier ND, et al. RET proto-oncogene: a review and update of genotype-phenotype correlations in hereditary medullary thyroid cancer and associated endocrine tumors. Thyroid. 2005;15:531–44.
21. Gagel RF, Levy ML, Donovan DT, et al. Multiple endocrine neoplasia type 2a associated with cutaneous lichen amyloidosis. Ann Intern Med. 1989;111:802–6.
22. Verdy M, Weber AM, Roy CC, et al. Hirschsprung's disease in a family with multiple endocrine neoplasia type 2. J Pediatr Gastroenterol Nutr. 1982;1:603–7.
23. Farndon JR, Leight GS, Dilley WG, et al. Familial medullary thyroid carcinoma without associated endocrinopathies: a distinct clinical entity. Br J Surg. 1986;73:278–81.

24. Eng C, Clayton D, Schuffenecker I, et al. The relationship between specific RET proto-oncogene mutations and disease phenotype in multiple endocrine neoplasia type 2. International RET mutation consortium analysis. JAMA. 1996;276:1575–9.

25. Elisei R, Romei C, Cosci B, et al. RET Genetic screening in patients with medullary thyroid cancer and their relatives: Experience with 807 individuals at one center. J Clin Endocrinol Metab. 2007;92:4725–9.

26. Carlson KM, Bracamontes J, Jackson CE, et al. Parent-of-origin effects in multiple endocrine neoplasia type 2B. Am J Hum Genet. 1994;55:1076–82.

27. Force ATAGT, Kloos RT, Eng C, Evans DB, et al. Medullary thyroid cancer: management guidelines of the American Thyroid Association. Thyroid. 2009;19:565–612.

28. Rosenthal M, Diekema D. Pediatric ethics guidelines for hereditary medullary thyroid cancer. Int J Pediatr Endocrinol. 2011;2011:847603.

29. Quayle FJ, Moley JF. Medullary thyroid carcinoma: management of lymph node metastases. Curr Treat Options Oncol. 2005;6:347–54.

30. Pacini F, Fontanelli M, Fugazzola L, et al. Routine measurement of serum calcitonin in nodular thyroid diseases allows the preoperative diagnosis of unsuspected sporadic medullary thyroid carcinoma. J Clin Endocrinol Metab. 1994;78:826–9.

31. Elisei R. Impact of routine measurement of serum calcitonin on the diagnosis and outcome of medullary thyroid cancer: experience in 10,864 patients with nodular thyroid disorders. J Clin Endocrinol Metab. 2004;89:163–8.

32. Gibelin H, Essique D, Jones C, et al. Increased calcitonin level in thyroid nodules without medullary carcinoma. Br J Surg. 2005;92:574–8.

33. Costante G, Meringolo D, Durante C, et al. Predictive value of serum calcitonin levels for pre-operative diagnosis of medullary thyroid carcinoma in a cohort of 5817 consecutive patients with thyroid nodules. J Clin Endocrinol Metab. 2006;92:450–5.

34. Daniels GH. Screening for medullary thyroid carcinoma with serum calcitonin measurements in patients with thyroid nodules in the United States and Canada. Thyroid. 2011;21:1199–207.

35. Colombo C, Verga U, Mian C, et al. Comparison of calcium and pentagastrin tests for the diagnosis and follow-up of medullary thyroid cancer. J Clin Endocrinol Metab. 2012;97:905–13.

36. Borget I, De Pouvourville G, Schlumberger M. Calcitonin determination in patients with nodular thyroid disease. J Clin Endocrinol Metab. 2006;92:425–7.

37. Cheung K, Roman SA, Wang TS, et al. Calcitonin measurement in the evaluation of thyroid nodules in the United States: a cost-effectiveness and decision analysis. J Clin Endocrinol Metab. 2008;93:2173–80.

38. Gharib H, Papini E, Paschke R, et al. American Association of Clinical Endocrinologists, Associazione Medici Endocrinologi, and European Thyroid Association Medical guidelines for clinical practice for the diagnosis and management of thyroid nodules: executive summary of recommendations. Endocr Pract. 2010;16:468–75.

39. Guerrero MA, Lindsay S, Suh I, et al. Medullary thyroid cancer: it is a pain in the neck? J Cancer. 2011;2:200–5.

40. Boi F, Maurelli I, Pinna G, et al. Calcitonin measurement in wash-out fluid from fine needle aspiration of neck masses in patients with primary and metastatic medullary thyroid carcinoma. J Clin Endocrinol Metab. 2007;92:2115–8.

41. Cohen R, Campos JM, Salaun C, et al. Preoperative calcitonin levels are predictive of tumor size and postoperative calcitonin normalization in medullary thyroid carcinoma. Groupe d'Etudes des Tumeurs a Calcitonine (GETC). J Clin Endocrinol Metab. 2000;85:919–22.

42. Machens A. Prospects of remission in medullary thyroid carcinoma according to basal calcitonin level. J Clin Endocrinol Metab. 2005;90:2029–34.

43. Machens A, Ukkat J, Hauptmann S, et al. Abnormal carcinoembryonic antigen levels and medullary thyroid cancer progression: a multivariate analysis. Arch Surg. 2007;142:289–93.

44. Blind E, Schmidt-Gayk H, Sinn HP, et al. Chromogranin A as tumor marker in medullary thyroid carcinoma. Thyroid. 1992;2:5–10.

45. Romei C, Cosci B, Renzini G, et al. RET genetic screening of sporadic medullary thyroid cancer (MTC) allows the preclinical diagnosis of unsuspected gene carriers and the identification of a relevant percentage of hidden familial MTC (FMTC). Clin Endocrinol. 2011;74:241–7.

46. Bugalho MJ, Domingues R, Santos JR, et al. Mutation analysis of the RET protooncogene and early thyroidectomy: results of a Portuguese cancer centre. Surgery. 2007;141:90–5.
47. Moley JF, DeBenedetti MK. Patterns of nodal metastases in palpable medullary thyroid carcinoma: recommendations for extent of node dissection. Ann Surg. 1999;229:880–7.
48. American Thyroid Association Surgery Working Group, American Association of Endocrine Surgeons, American Academy of Otolaryngology-Head and Neck Surgery, American Head and Neck Society, Carty SE, Cooper DS, et al. Consensus statement on the terminology and classification of central neck dissection for thyroid cancer. Thyroid. 2009;19:1153–8.
49. de Groot JWB, Links TP, Sluiter WJ, et al. Locoregional control in patients with palpable medullary thyroid cancer: results of standardized compartment-oriented surgery. Head Neck. 2007;29:857–63.
50. Scollo C. Rationale for central and bilateral lymph node dissection in sporadic and hereditary medullary thyroid cancer. J Clin Endocrinol Metab. 2003;88:2070–5.
51. Machens A, Hauptmann S, Dralle H. Increased risk of lymph node metastasis in multifocal hereditary and sporadic medullary thyroid cancer. World J Surg. 2007;31:1960–5.
52. Kazaure HS, Roman SA, Sosa JA. Medullary thyroid microcarcinoma. Cancer. 2011;118:620–7.
53. Machens A, Hauptmann S, Dralle H. Prediction of lateral lymph node metastases in medullary thyroid cancer. Br J Surg. 2008;95:586–91.
54. Kebebew E, Ituarte PH, Siperstein AE, et al. Medullary thyroid carcinoma: clinical characteristics, treatment, prognostic factors, and a comparison of staging systems. Cancer. 2000;88:1139–48.
55. Dralle H, Damm I, Scheumann GF, et al. Frequency and significance of cervicomediastinal lymph node metastases in medullary thyroid carcinoma: results of a compartment-oriented microdissection method. Henry Ford Hosp Med J. 1992;40:264–7.
56. Machens A, Holzhausen H-J, Dralle H. Contralateral cervical and mediastinal lymph node metastasis in medullary thyroid cancer: systemic disease? Surgery. 2006;139:28–32.
57. Tung WS, Vesely TM, Moley JF. Laparoscopic detection of hepatic metastases in patients with residual or recurrent medullary thyroid cancer. Surgery. 1995;118:1024–9; discussion 1029–30.
58. Edge SB, Byrd DR, Compton CC, editors. AJCC cancer staging manual. 7th ed. New York: Springer; 2010.
59. Modigliani E, Cohen R, Campos JM, et al. Prognostic factors for survival and for biochemical cure in medullary thyroid carcinoma: results in 899 patients. The GETC Study Group. Groupe d'etude des tumeurs a calcitonine. Clin Endocrinol (Oxf). 1998;48:265–73.
60. Pelizzo MR, Boschin IM, Bernante P, et al. Natural history, diagnosis, treatment and outcome of medullary thyroid cancer: 37 years experience on 157 patients. Eur J Surg Oncol. 2007;33:493–7.
61. Bhattacharyya N. A population-based analysis of survival factors in differentiated and medullary thyroid carcinoma. Otolaryngol Head Neck Surg. 2003;128:115–23.
62. Roman S, Lin R, Sosa JA. Prognosis of medullary thyroid carcinoma. Cancer. 2006;107:2134–42.
63. Ahmed SR, Ball DW. Incidentally discovered medullary thyroid cancer: diagnostic strategies and treatment. J Clin Endocrinol Metab. 2011;96:1237–45.
64. Valle LA, Kloos RT. The prevalence of occult medullary thyroid carcinoma at autopsy. J Clin Endocrinol Metab. 2011;96:E109–13.
65. Davidson BJ, Burman KD. Cancer of the thyroid and parathyroid. In: Harrison LB, Sessions RB, Hong WK, editors. Head and neck cancer: a multidisciplinary approach. 3rd ed. Philadelphia: Lippincott Williams & Wilkins; 2008. p. 992.
66. Yip DT, Hassan M, Pazaitou-Panayiotou K, et al. Preoperative basal calcitonin and tumor stage correlate with postoperative calcitonin normalization in patients undergoing initial surgical management of medullary thyroid carcinoma. Surgery. 2011;150:1168–77.
67. Machens A, Gimm O, Ukkat J, et al. Improved prediction of calcitonin normalization in medullary thyroid carcinoma patients by quantitative lymph node analysis. Cancer. 2000;88:1909–15.
68. Pellegriti G, Leboulleux S, Baudin E, et al. Long-term outcome of medullary thyroid carcinoma in patients with normal postoperative medical imaging. Br J Cancer. 2003;88:1537–42.
69. Franc S, Niccoli-Sire P, Cohen R, et al. Complete surgical lymph node resection does not prevent authentic recurrences of medullary thyroid carcinoma. Clin Endocrinol. 2001;55:403–9.

70. Miyauchi A, Onishi T, Morimoto S, et al. Relation of doubling time of plasma calcitonin levels to prognosis and recurrence of medullary thyroid carcinoma. Ann Surg. 1984;199:461–6.
71. Gawlik T, d'Amico A, Szpak-Ulczok S, et al. The prognostic value of tumor markers doubling times in medullary thyroid carcinoma-preliminary report. Thyroid Res. 2010;3:10.
72. Barbet J. Prognostic impact of serum calcitonin and carcinoembryonic antigen doubling times in patients with medullary thyroid carcinoma. J Clin Endocrinol Metab. 2005;90:6077–84.
73. Meijer JAA, le Cessie S, van den Hout WB, et al. Calcitonin and carcinoembryonic antigen doubling times as prognostic factors in medullary thyroid carcinoma: a structured meta-analysis. Clin Endocrinol. 2010;72:534–42.
74. Busnardo B, Girelli ME, Simioni N, et al. Nonparallel patterns of calcitonin and carcinoembryonic antigen levels in the follow-up of medullary thyroid carcinoma. Cancer. 1984;53:278–85.
75. Fialkowski E, DeBenedetti M, Moley J. Long-term outcome of reoperations for medullary thyroid carcinoma. World J Surg. 2008;32:754–65.
76. Giraudet AL, Vanel D, Lebolleux S, et al. Imaging medullary thyroid carcinoma with persistent elevated calcitonin levels. J Clin Endocrinol Metab. 2007;92:4185–90.
77. Ong SC, Schoder H, Patel SG, et al. Diagnostic accuracy of 18F-FDG PET in restaging patients with medullary thyroid carcinoma and elevated calcitonin levels. J Nucl Med. 2007;48:501–7.
78. Treglia G, Castaldi P, Villani MF, et al. Comparison of 18F-DOPA, 18F-FDG and 68Ga-somatostatin analogue PET/CT in patients with recurrent medullary thyroid carcinoma. Eur J Nucl Med Mol Imaging. 2012;39:569–80.
79. Beheshti M, Pocher S, Vali R, et al. The value of 18F-DOPA PET-CT in patients with medullary thyroid carcinoma: Comparison with 18F-FDG PET-CT. Eur Radiol. 2009;19:1425–34.
80. Kauhanen S, Schalin-Jantti C, Seppanen M, et al. Complementary roles of 18F-DOPA PET/CT and 18F-FDG PET/CT in medullary thyroid cancer. J Nucl Med. 2011;52:1855–63.
81. Naswa N, Sharma P, Suman Kc S, et al. Prospective evaluation of 68Ga-DOTANOC PET-CT in patients with recurrent medullary thyroid carcinoma. Nucl Med Commun. 2012;33:766–74.
82. Conry BG, Papathanasiou ND, Prakash V, et al. Comparison of (68)Ga-DOTATATE and (18) F-fluorodeoxyglucose PET/CT in the detection of recurrent medullary thyroid carcinoma. Eur J Nucl Med Mol Imaging. 2010;37:49–57.
83. Lodish M, Dagalakis U, Chen CC, et al. ^{111}In-Octreotide scintigraphy for identification of metastatic medullary thyroid carcinoma in children and adolescents. J Clin Endocrinol Metab. 2012;97:E207–12.
84. Tisell LE, Hansson G, Jansson S, et al. Reoperation in the treatment of asymptomatic metastasizing medullary thyroid carcinoma. Surgery. 1986;99:60–6.
85. Moley JF, Dilley WG, DeBenedetti MK. Improved results of cervical reoperation for medullary thyroid carcinoma. Ann Surg. 1997;225:734–40.
86. van Heerden JA, Grant CS, Gharib H, et al. Long-term course of patients with persistent hypercalcitoninemia after apparent curative primary surgery for medullary thyroid carcinoma. Ann Surg. 1990;212:395–400.
87. Moley JF, DeBenedetti MK, Dilley WG, et al. Surgical management of patients with persistent or recurrent medullary thyroid cancer. J Intern Med. 1998;243:521–6.
88. Schwartz DL, Rana V, Shaw S, et al. Postoperative radiotherapy for advanced medullary thyroid cancer—local disease control in the modern era. Head Neck. 2008;30:883–8.
89. Terezakis SA, Lee KS, Ghossein RA, et al. Role of external beam radiotherapy in patients with advanced or recurrent nonanaplastic thyroid cancer: Memorial Sloan-Kettering Cancer Center experience. Int J Radiat Oncol Biol Phys. 2009;73:795–801.
90. Fife KM, Bower M, Harmer CL. Medullary thyroid cancer: the role of radiotherapy in local control. Eur J Surg Oncol. 1996;22:588–91.
91. Brierley J, Tsang R, Simpson WJ, et al. Medullary thyroid cancer: analyses of survival and prognostic factors and the role of radiation therapy in local control. Thyroid. 1996;6:305–10.
92. Martinez SR, Beal SH, Chen A, et al. Adjuvant external beam radiation for medullary thyroid carcinoma. J Surg Oncol. 2010;102:175–8.

93. Wells SA, Robinson BG, Gagel RF, et al. Vandetanib in patients with locally advanced or metastatic medullary thyroid cancer: a randomized, double-blind phase III trial. J Clin Oncol. 2012;30:134–41.

94. Chatal JF. Survival improvement in patients with medullary thyroid carcinoma who undergo pretargeted anti-carcinoembryonic-antigen radioimmunotherapy: a collaborative study with the French Endocrine Tumor Group. J Clin Oncol. 2006;24:1705–11.

95. Salaun P-Y, Campion L, Bournaud C, et al. Phase II trial of anticarcinoembryonic antigen pretargeted radioimmunotherapy in progressive metastatic medullary thyroid carcinoma: biomarker response and survival improvement. J Nucl Med. 2012;53:1185–92.

96. Iten F, Muller B, Schindler C, et al. Response to [^{90}Yttrium-DOTA]-TOC treatment is associated with long-term survival benefit in metastasized medullary thyroid cancer: a phase II clinical trial. Clin Cancer Res. 2007;13:6696–702.

97. Castellani MR, Seregni E, Maccauro M, et al. MIBG for diagnosis and therapy of medullary thyroid carcinoma: is there still a role? Q J Nucl Med Mol Imaging. 2008;52:430–40.

98. Pasieka JL, McEwan AJB, Rorstad O. The palliative role of ^{131}I-MIBG and ^{111}In-octreotide therapy in patients with metastatic progressive neuroendocrine neoplasms. Surgery. 2004;136:1218–26.

99. Mahler C, Verhelst J, de Longueville M, et al. Long-term treatment of metastatic medullary thyroid carcinoma with the somatostatin analogue octreotide. Clin Endocrinol. 1990;33:261–9.

100. Chen H, Roberts JR, Ball DW, et al. Effective long-term palliation of symptomatic, incurable metastatic medullary thyroid cancer by operative resection. Ann Surg. 1998;227:887–95.

101. Akyildiz HY, Mitchell J, Milas M, et al. Laparoscopic radiofrequency thermal ablation of neuroendocrine hepatic metastases: long-term follow-up. Surgery. 2010;148:1288–93.

102. Lorenz K, Brauckhoff M, Behrmann C, et al. Selective arterial chemoembolization for hepatic metastases from medullary thyroid carcinoma. Surgery. 2005;138:986–93.

103. Fromigue J. Chemoembolization for liver metastases from medullary thyroid carcinoma. J Clin Endocrinol Metab. 2006;91:2496–9.

Anaplastic Thyroid Cancer: Current Concepts

9

Sylvie Galindo and Sam M. Wiseman

Introduction

ATC is one of the most aggressive and lethal human malignancies. It is rare, accounting for <2 % of thyroid cancers [1–3], but it is the cause of a disproportionate (14–50 %) number of thyroid cancer-related deaths [3, 4]. The prognosis for individuals diagnosed with ATC is poor; the median survival is short (3–5 months after diagnosis), and long-term survival is unusual [3, 5–7]. Population-based reports on North American patients cite a 13–14 % 10-year survival rate [1, 3]. A study from Slovenia had a 6 % 2-year survival rate [8], and a study from Japan reported 0 % survival at 5 years [4]. These observations are in stark contrast to the highly favourable prognosis for the more commonly diagnosed differentiated types of thyroid cancer [3, 9].

Similar to all other thyroid cancer types, ATC affects women (male gender prognostic factor for WDTC, as stated in Chaps. 2, 6, and 7) more commonly than men [3, 5, 6, 10] and ATC is most commonly diagnosed in the elderly, with the median age at diagnosis being higher than that for other types of thyroid cancer [2, 10]. One group found that 67 % of individuals diagnosed with ATC were >70 years of age [2]. A North American study demonstrated additional variance in the incidence of ATC in different racial and ethnic groups [10]. Among women, ATC rates were highest among Hispanics, and among men, Asians were more frequently diagnosed with ATC [10]. According to a retrospective cohort study carried out by Davies and Welch, the incidence of ATC has not changed significantly between 1973 and 2002, despite an increase in the incidence of thyroid cancer during the same time period [11]. The average size of the tumour at diagnosis of ATCs has decreased over the

S. Galindo • S.M. Wiseman (✉)
Department of Surgery, St. Paul's Hospital & University of British Columbia,
C303–1081 Burrard Street, Vancouver, BC V6Z 1Y6, Canada
e-mail: smwiseman@providencehealth.bc.ca

© K. Alok Pathak, Richard W. Nason, Janice L. Pasieka, Rehan Kazi,
Raghav C. Dwivedi 2015
Springer India/Byword Books
K.A. Pathak et al. (eds.), *Management of Thyroid Cancer: Special Considerations*,
Head and Neck Cancer Clinics, DOI 10.1007/978-81-322-2434-1_9

113

past two decades; the smaller ATC tumour size is associated with an improved long-term survival [12]. Several patient factors have been found to influence the prognosis of individuals diagnosed with ATC. Younger age at diagnosis is a favourable prognostic factor, and significantly higher survival rates have been reported in patients in the following age groups: (i) <45 years [3], (ii) <60 years [5], and (iii) <65 years [13]. Female gender, intrathyroidal tumour extent [5, 8], lack of distant metastases at diagnosis [7], and higher patient performance status, according to the Eastern Cooperative Oncology Group scale [8], also predict a better disease prognosis. Sugitani et al. devised a prognostic index based on four characteristics that were associated with a decreased survival in ATC patients [14]. The factors included in their prognostic index were: (i) presence of acute symptoms (hoarseness, neck pain, dyspnoea, dysphagia, rapidly growing neck mass), (ii) leukocytosis ($\geq$10,000/mm [3]), (iii) tumour size of >5 cm, and (iv) the presence of distant metastasis [14]. This index was then prospectively validated in a group of 74 ATC patients. Six-month survival rates were found to be significantly lower in patients who had 3 or more of these 4 prognostic factors, compared to patients with one or none of these prognostic factors, and were 12 % and 72 %, respectively [15]. A report based on the SEER (Surveillance, Epidemiology and End Results) database found that the median survival of ATC patients was 9 months when the cancer was confined to the thyroid, 6 months if adjacent structures were involved, and 3 months in the presence of distant metastases [16]. The 1-year survival rates for ATC in this report were 50 %, 27.6 % and 7.4 %, respectively [16].

Clinical Presentation

According to the current American Joint Committee on Cancer (AJCC) staging system for thyroid cancer, al! individuals diagnosed with ATC are classified as having stage IV disease. Disease limited to the thyroid is classified as stage IVA, extrathyroidal extension defines stage IVB, and disease associated with distant metastasis is considered stage IVC. Locoregional lymph node involvement may be present in stages IVA and IVB. A recent review found that the median proportion of patients presenting with stage IVA, IVB and IVC disease was 10.2 %, 40.2 % and 45.8 %, respectively [17]. One study reported 98 % of ATCs to be locally invasive at the time of their diagnosis [6].

Individuals diagnosed with ATC have been found to be more likely to have a history of an enlarging thyroid mass, or presumed goitre, before their diagnosis (25 % vs. 14.3 % for papillary thyroid cancer [PTC] and 15.9 % for follicular thyroid cancer [FTC]), as well as a history of head and neck exposure to radiation (9.4 % vs. 4.7 % for all types of thyroid cancer) [2]. Coexisting thyroid pathology is common in individuals diagnosed with ATC, including DTC and multinodular goitre [5]. ATC patients tend to present with larger tumours than patients with other types of thyroid cancer. The median tumour size at diagnosis in one report was 50 mm for ATC, 17 mm for PTC, 30 mm for FTC, 35 mm for Hürthle cell carcinoma (HCC), 28 mm for familial medullary thyroid cancer (MTC), and 8 mm for sporadic MTC [2].

Not surprisingly, as they tend to present with advanced disease, ATC patients are more likely to be symptomatic at the time of diagnosis than patients with other types of thyroid cancer. Local symptoms caused by mass effect and local invasion from the cancer, including dysphagia (in 40 % of patients), hoarseness or voice changes (40.6 %), and stridor (24 %) are most common at presentation. Other common findings at disease presentation include neck pain (26 %) and the presence of a regional lymph node mass (54.2 %) [2]. As already discussed, the presence of acute symptoms predicts a shorter survival for ATC patients [14, 15]. A report evaluating the cause of death in fatal cases of thyroid cancer found the following aetiologies for individuals succumbing to ATC: (i) respiratory insufficiency (40.6 %), (ii) circulatory failure (16.2 %), (iii) haemorrhage from tumour (13.5 %), (iv) airway obstruction (16.2 %), and (v) other causes, which include sepsis, disseminated intravascular coagulopathy, renal failure and hypercalcaemia (13.5 %) [4]. Respiratory insufficiency developed from the replacement of large volumes of lung tissue by pulmonary metastases in most patients, while circulatory failure was caused by cardiac failure, vena caval compression and cardiac metastasis. Deaths from airway obstruction resulting from stenosis, vocal cord oedema and asphyxia were more frequent in ATC patients who did not undergo a tracheostomy [4].

When clinically suspected, it is important to establish a diagnosis of ATC expeditiously in order to organize a timely therapeutic approach for this aggressive cancer [17]. ATC diagnosis requires sampling of the tumour through fine-needle aspiration (FNA) or core biopsy. For cases in which FNA or core biopsy yield non-diagnostic material, it is recommended to proceed with open biopsy to confirm the diagnosis of ATC and rule out a less aggressive tumour [17]. Histological analysis might reveal one or more of a variety of histological subtypes of ATC, viz. spindle cell, giant cell and squamoid cell. The ATC histological subtype generally does not predict disease prognosis. Imaging studies, including CT, ultrasound and magnetic resonance imaging, are important at the time of diagnosis of ATC for evaluating the locoregional spread of disease, as well as to identify distant metastasis [17]. In addition, every patient should undergo initial assessment of the vocal cords with fibreoptic laryngoscopy or mirror examination [17].

Molecular and Genetic Characteristics

Anaplastic Transformation

ATC is believed to arise from or 'transform' from pre-existing DTC. This belief is based upon clinical, pathological and molecular evidence [18]. Whether this postmalignant thyroid cancer progression is responsible for all cases of ATC, or if some ATCs arise de novo, is unknown.

The observation that ATC may occur in older people with a prior or concurrent history of DTC suggested that ATC may somehow be related to DTC. Furthermore, individuals who have a DTC component associated with their anaplastic tumour seem to have a better prognosis [19]. The observation that ATCs have tended to be a smaller size at the time of their diagnosis, along with the increase in the observed frequency of coexistent DTC with ATC over the past two decades, lends further clinical support to ATC arising from DTC [12].

Between 23 and 90 % of ATCs contain foci of DTC on pathological analysis (PTC in most cases, as well as FTC and HCC reported). Histological transition zones have also been identified between the two distinct thyroid tumour components. These areas show greater nuclear atypia and architectural distortion than the associated DTC foci [18].

Comparison of inter-simple sequence repeat polymerase chain reaction products from adjacent foci of PTC and ATC has shown shared genomic alterations [20]. Evidence also exists that suggests PTCs that contain a mutated BRAF gene are more prone to undergo anaplastic transformation [21]. The BRAF oncogene is present in 20–69 % of PTC, and is associated with uncontrolled cellular proliferation and a worse disease prognosis [21]. Several studies have shown that ATCs that have a BRAF mutation contain foci of PTC that share the same mutated sequence on genomic analysis [21–23]. Specific shared N–RAS mutations have also been identified in ATC and FTC components of the same tumours [23].

Mutations in TP53 have been found in the ATC but not in the PTC components of anaplastic tumours, suggesting that p53 is involved in the progression from high-risk, *BRAF*-mutated PTC to ATC. Additionally, ATCs have been found to harbour significantly larger chromosomal alterations than PTCs, suggesting that the aggressiveness of the tumour is related to the extent of its genetic alterations [24].

Molecular Alterations

A variety of important cellular functions and pathways have been found to be altered in ATC compared to DTC. In a study reported by our group, thyroglobulin, Bcl-2, MIB-1, E-cadherin, and p53 were significantly differentially expressed in ATC and adjacent coexisting DTC [25].

ATC cells overexpress epidermal growth factor receptor (EGFR) both in vitro and in vivo, making EGFR a promising drug target for the treatment of ATC. Evidence from in vitro and mouse studies suggests that gefitinib may halt cellular proliferation and induce apoptosis in ATC by blocking the activation of EGFR [26]. A recent study showed that inhibition of EGFR and vascular endothelial growth factor receptor 2 (VEGFR2) with vandetanib slowed ATC cell-line growth in a murine model [27].

Therapeutic Approach

Despite progress in understanding and treating human cancer, the prognosis for ATC has remained dismal. The most promising treatment strategies for ATC are multimodal, incorporating combinations of surgery, radiotherapy and chemotherapy [13, 16, 28–31].

Surgery

Unlike other forms of thyroid cancer, surgery is rarely curative for ATC. The type of operation and the extent of resection, if any, vary among ATC patients and depend on their extent of disease at presentation. Not only is surgical resection rarely curative, it may also lead to significant morbidity because of large tumour size, locoregional tumour extension into important structures that include the trachea, oesophagus and spine, and the presence of distant metastases at diagnosis. Indeed, compared to DTC, for which complete surgical resection with no residual tumour (R0) is achieved in the majority of cases (68–88.5 %) depending upon histology, an R0 resection is only achieved in 8.7 % of ATC cases [2]. Furthermore, residual microscopic tumour is left in 12 % of cases, and residual macroscopic tumour is not removed in 23.9 % of surgically managed ATC cases [2]. Patients who require total thyroidectomy with selective or radical lymph node dissection for cancer have higher rates of postoperative complications than patients who undergo more limited resections (i.e. partial thyroidectomy or total thyroidectomy without lymph node dissection). Specifically, airway problems, bleeding, hypocalcaemia, recurrent laryngeal nerve dysfunction and wound infections are more common with more radical operations [2].

Evidence suggests that preoperative radiation therapy and neoadjuvant chemotherapy may lead to a reduction in the extent of surgery that is required for ATC, making total thyroidectomy and neck dissection only necessary for some cases [32]. Neoadjuvant radiotherapy and/or chemotherapy may be given in cases deemed to be unresectable in order to reduce tumour bulk and potentially allow for delayed primary resection [17]. Curative resection (R0/R1) and surgical reduction of tumour bulk (R2) before chemotherapy or radiotherapy may increase their effectiveness and has been shown to improve survival in ATC patients [33–35]. Surgical control of local disease may also obviate the need for palliative tracheostomy in these patients [34]. Many questions remain regarding the timing of surgery, its extent, and the role of tracheostomy in the management of ATC.

Some evidence suggests that higher preoperative radiation doses might be associated with improved outcomes when compared to lower preoperative doses given in conjunction with postoperative radiation [29]. The results of a recent systematic review suggest that the surgical treatment of cervical lymph node metastases may have little effect on disease prognosis, possibly because of the disproportionately greater importance of other ATC patient factors [34]. Evidence supports the observation that longer survival and lower morbidity are achieved in ATC patients with surgical resection aimed at controlling local disease when compared to prophylactic tracheostomy, followed by radiation and chemotherapy [36]. Generally, it is recommended that tracheostomy be employed as a treatment for impending airway obstruction and not as a prophylactic surgical measure [17, 34].

Radiotherapy

Combined surgical resection and radiotherapy has been shown to reduce cause-specific mortality in ATC patients when compared to surgery alone [5, 16, 35].

A study of 261 ATC patients treated with a combination of surgery and radiotherapy found that the addition of radiation led to improved survival of patients with disease extending into adjacent structures, but not for patients with intracapsular disease or distant metastases [16]. It is recommended that patients begin adjuvant radiotherapy as soon as they have sufficiently recovered from surgical resection, which usually happens 2 or 3 weeks postoperatively [17].

In particular, higher doses of radiation (>45 Gy) have been shown to improve survival in ATC patients when compared to lower doses [35]. Another study showed that patients without distant metastases who were receiving ≥50 Gy had superior survival [37]. However, toxicity becomes a concern when high radiation doses are employed. In ATC patients who received doses of radiation of ≥50 Gy, the complications included: (i) hospitalization for dehydration, (ii) need for acute airway management, (iii) pneumonia during treatment, and (iv) development of chronic oesophageal stricture after treatment completion. Twenty-three per cent of ATC patients who received radiation therapy developed complications, and the rate did not differ significantly in patients who underwent 3-dimensional radiotherapy compared to patients who underwent intensity-modulated radiotherapy (IMRT) [37].

Chemotherapy

The addition of radiosensitizing adjuvant chemotherapy to surgical resection and IMRT in ATC patients has been found to improve survival in patients with stage IVA and stage IVB disease [31]. The 1-year and 2-year survival rates in the study by Foote et al. were 70 % and 60 %, respectively [31]. The role of chemotherapy in the presence of IVC disease is less clear.

A small retrospective study suggested that the combination of radiotherapy (≤60 Gy) and docetaxel led to complete remission in 4 of 6 patients at a median follow-up of 21.5 months; however, this was associated with substantial treatment-related toxicities [38]. In another report, patients who underwent surgery that was followed by doxorubicin, cisplatin and radiation therapy had a 3-year survival rate of 27 % [30]. However, acute toxicities that included pharyngo-oesophagitis, neutropenia, thrombocytopenia and anaemia were observed in 33 %, 73 %, 13 % and 27 % of cases, respectively [30].

Two recent studies of ATC patient cohorts treated with a combination of surgery, radiotherapy and chemotherapy yielded promising results. Derbel et al. reported on 44 ATC patients who underwent total thyroidectomy and cervical lymph node dissection followed by doxorubicin, cisplastin and 46–50 Gy of hyperfractionated radiation [28]. Fourteen of 44 patients (32 %) had a complete response and the median survival observed in this study was 7 months. Tennvall et al. reported a study of 55 ATC patients in which three different treatment protocols were used [29]. Patients receiving the full dose of radiation preoperatively and doxorubicin postoperatively had the best outcomes, with no sign of local recurrence in 17 of 22 patients (77 %). The other two protocol groups received smaller doses of radiation both preoperatively and postoperatively, while the remainder of their treatment was the same [29].

Evidence indicates that induction chemotherapy with weekly paclitaxel is effective in improving survival in individuals diagnosed with stage IVB ATC, compared to other types of chemotherapy [39]. However, patients with stage IVC disease do not benefit [39]. The current American Thyroid Association guidelines recommend that patients with non-metastatic ATC undergo some combination of taxane (paclitaxel or docetaxel), and/ or anthracyclines (doxorubicin), and/or platin (cisplatin or carboplatin) chemotherapy in addition to radiotherapy [17]. This should be initiated as soon as the patient has sufficiently recovered postoperatively [17].

Targeted Molecular Therapies and Future Directions

Selective tyrosine kinase (TK) inhibitors have been shown to retard the growth of ATC cell lines in vitro and in vivo [26, 27, 40, 41]. Gleevec® [Novartis Pharmaceuticals Corporation, East Hanover, New Jersey] in combination with radiotherapy, has been shown to inhibit ATC tumour growth more than either treatment alone in a murine model [41]. Imatinib and gefitinib have also been shown to enhance apoptosis of ATC cell lines in vitro and in vivo in a mouse model [40]. The two drugs in combination have greater antitumour activity than each drug alone [40]. Imatinib has also been shown to enhance the induction of ATC cell apoptosis by docetaxel [42].

A small clinical trial of patients with advanced ATC (locoregional or metastatic disease) showed that imatinib had some activity and tolerable toxicities [43]. Of 8 patients, 2 had a partial response, as measured on imaging, whereas 4 showed stable disease at 8 weeks after the initiation of treatment [43]. Pazopanib, an inhibitor of kinases, including VEGFR, showed promise as an agent against ATC in a xenograft model [44]. However, in a multicentre clinical trial, it did not produce a RECIST (response evaluation criteria in solid tumours) response in ATC patients treated with this agent in isolation [44].

Several molecular targets show promise as therapeutic candidates for ATC treatment. Chrysin, a potential notch inducer, was shown to inhibit the growth of ATC by inducing apoptosis both in vitro and in a xenograft tumour model [45]. A replication-competent vaccinia virus with oncolytic activity was used to infect ATC cell lines in vitro. The vaccinia virus displayed cytotoxic activity against the ATC cells, proving to be a promising avenue of treatment that warranted further investigation [46]. Metalloprotinease-activated anthrax lethal toxin has shown potential as a mitogen-activated TK pathway inhibitor in vitro. A study using a mouse model that contained an ATC cell line xenograft showed the ability of this toxin to inhibit tumour progression [47]. Recently, our group has reviewed the growing literature on targeted therapy for treatment of ATC [48].

Summary

ATC is an uncommon and aggressive thyroid malignancy. Whereas it accounts for only 2 % of all thyroid cancer cases, it is responsible for ≤50 % of the mortality attributed to thyroid cancer. It is primarily a disease of the elderly, with most patients being diagnosed over the age of 65 years.

All ATCs are considered to be stage IV disease when classified by the current AJCC staging system. Stage IVA represents intrathyroidal disease, IVB locoregional spread and IVC distant metastasis. ATC usually presents with a rapidly growing neck mass and many patients have symptoms attributable to the tumour at presentation, including dyspnoea, dysphagia and voice changes. The median proportion of patients presenting with distant metastasis is 45.8 %, and disease prognosis is affected negatively by greater extent of disease at presentation, as well as patient factors, including leukocytosis ($\geq$10,000/mm [3]), acute symptoms at diagnosis, tumour size of >5 cm, and the presence of distant metastasis.

ATC is believed to arise through anaplastic transformation of DTC and clinical, pathological and molecular evidence supports this intratumoral evolutionary process.

Treatment of ATC has remained largely ineffective, and the disease is almost uniformly fatal. Multimodal therapy has shown promise, with various combinations of anticancer agents, radiotherapy and surgery yielding the best results. Promising new therapies, including targeted molecular treatments, such as selective TK inhibitors, show promise and warrant further investigation.

Commentary

Janice L. Pasieka

Anaplastic thyroid cancer (ATC) is a rare but highly lethal form of thyroid cancer. All ATCs are considered stage IV tumours, according to the current American Joint Committee on Cancer (AJCC) staging system. Galindo and Wiseman have provided strong evidence to suggest that an ATC develops from pre-existing well-differentiated thyroid cancer. The current treatment regimes are multimodal and include surgery, radiation and systemic therapy. This chapter covers presentation, the molecular and genetic characterization of these tumours, and the treatment option currently utilized. Although to date treatment of ATC remains largely ineffective, the authors outline the potential benefit of surgery, radiation, chemotherapy, and the newer targeted molecular therapies that have shown promise as therapeutic options.

Recently, guidelines for the management of ATC were published by the American Thyroid Association (ATA) [1]. This is the first time the ATA has put together guidelines for the management of ATC. This chapter nevertheless serves as a great resource for the clinician caring for patients with this rare tumour. To summarize, the ATA guidelines, patients with stages IVa and IVb (potentially resectable disease) should be treated with a multimodality approach, including surgery, external beam radiation and systemic therapy. The role of surgery in this disease ultimately depends on the disease characteristics. Ten per cent of patients with ATC present with intra-thyroidal disease alone. The recommendation from the ATA is for a total thyroidec-tomy with therapeutic lymph node dissection in these patients. When extrathyroidal is encountered, en bloc resection should be considered if grossly negative margins can be achieved. This is then followed by radiation and chemotherapy. Where sur-gery is not amenable as a first-line option, radiation and chemotherapy may down-stage the disease, allowing for surgery to aid with locoregional control.

Unresectable ATC patients may respond initially to systemic therapy in combi-nation with external beam radiation as such, patients with stage IVc disease (distant metastatic disease) should be considered for clinical trial or palliative care.

Systemic therapy, both targeted and with cytotoxic agents, has not shown clear benefits in improving survival or quality of life. Consequently, the need for the development of novel systemic therapeutic options is critical. As such, all patients with ATC should be considered for a therapeutic trial. The largest prospective study conducted in ATC was recently published [2]. The addition of fosbretabulin (CA4P), a novel tubulin-blinding compound, in combination with thyroid surgery, suggested an improvement in patient survival [2]. This FACT1 trial was a randomized con-trolled phase II/III trial assessed in the safety and efficacy of carboplatin/pacli-taxel—with or without CA4P. Unfortunately, the study was terminated after enrolling only 80 patients because of the low accrual rate of the subjects needed for the trial. This study illustrated the difficulty in enrolling patients with rare tumours across 40 centres in 11 different countries. However, it did provide insight into the need for multimodality therapy and the role surgery plays in this disease.

References

1. Smallridge RC, Ain KB, Asa SL, et al. American Thyroid Association guide-lines for the management of patients with anaplastic thyroid cancer. Thyroid. 2012;22:1104–39.

2. Sosa JA, Balkissoon J, Lu SP, et al. Thyroidectomy followed by fosbretabulin (CA4P) combination regimen appears to suggest improvement in patients survival in anaplastic thyroid cancer. Surgery. 2012;152:1078–87.

References

1. Gilliland FD, Hunt WC, Morris DM, et al. Prognostic factors for thyroid carcinoma: a population-based study of 15,698 cases from the surveillance, epidemiology and end results (SEER) Program 1973–1991. Cancer. 1997;79:564.
2. Hundahl SA, Blake C, Cunningham MP, et al. Initial results from a prospective cohort study of 5583 cases of thyroid carcinoma treated in the United States during 1996. Cancer. 2000;89:202.
3. Hundahl SA, Fleming ID, Fremgen AM, et al. A national cancer database report on 53,856 cases of thyroid carcinoma treated in the United States, 1985–1995. Cancer. 1998;83:2638–48.
4. Kitamura Y, Shimizu K, Nagahama M, et al. Immediate causes of death in thyroid carcinoma: clinicopathological analysis of 161 fatal cases. J Clin Endocrinol Metab. 1999;84:4043.
5. Kebebew E, Greenspan FS, Clark OH, et al. Anaplastic thyroid carcinoma treatment outcomes and prognostic factors. Cancer. 2005;103:1330.

6. McIver B, Hay ID, Giuffrida DF, et al. Anaplastic thyroid carcinoma: a 50-year experience at a single institution. Surgery. 2001;130:1028.
7. Segerhammar I, Larsson C, Nilsson I, et al. Anaplastic carcinoma of the thyroid gland: treatment and outcome over 13 years at one institution. J Surg Oncol. 2012;106:981–6.
8. Besic N, Hocevar M, Zgajnar J, et al. Prognostic factors in anaplastic carcinoma of the thyroid—a multivariate survival analysis of 188 patients. Lagenbecks Arch Surg. 2005;390:203.
9. Davies L, Welch HG. Thyroid cancer survival in the United States observational data from 1973 to 2005. Arch Otolaryngol Head Neck Surg. 2010;136:440.
10. Aschebrooke-Kilfoy B, Ward MH, Sabra MM, et al. Thyroid cancer incidence patterns in the United States by histologic type, 1992–2006. Thyroid. 2011;21:125.
11. Davies L, Welch HG. Increasing incidence of thyroid cancer in the United States, 1973–2002. JAMA. 2006;295:2164.
12. Han JM, Kim WB, Kim TY, et al. Time trend in tumour size and characteristics of anaplastic thyroid carcinoma. Clin Endocrinol. 2012;77:459.
13. Yau T, Lo CY, Epstein RJ, et al. Treatment outcomes in anaplastic thyroid carcinoma: survival improvement in young patients with localized disease treated by combination of surgery and radiotherapy. Ann Surg Oncol. 2008;15:2500.
14. Sugitani I, Kasai N, Fujimoto Y, et al. Prognostic factors and therapeutic strategy for anaplastic carcinoma of the thyroid. World J Surg. 2001;25:617.
15. Orita Y, Sugitani I, Amemiya T, et al. Prospective application of our novel prognostic index in the treatment of anaplastic thyroid carcinoma. Surgery. 2011;150:1212.
16. Chen J, Tward JD, Shrieve DC, et al. Surgery and radiotherapy improves survival in patients with anaplastic thyroid carcinoma analysis of surveillance, epidemiology, and end results 1983–2002. Am J Clin Oncol. 2008;31:460.
17. Smallridge RC. Approach to the patient with anaplastic thyroid carcinoma. J Clin Endocrinol Metab. 2012;97:2566.
18. Wiseman SM, Loree TR, Rigual NR, et al. Anaplastic transformation of thyroid cancer: review of clinical, pathologic, and molecular evidence provides new insights into disease biology and future therapy. Head Neck. 2003;25:662.
19. Rodriguez JM, Pinero A, Ortiz S, et al. Clinical and histological differences in anaplastic thyroid carcinoma. Eur J Surg. 2000;166:34–8.
20. Wiseman SM, Loree TR, Hicks WL, et al. Anaplastic thyroid cancer evolved from papillary carcinoma. Arch Otolaryngol Head Neck Surg. 2003;129:96.
21. Gauchotte G, Phillipe C, Lacomme S, et al. BRAF, p53, and SOX2 in anaplastic thyroid carcinoma: evidence for multistep carcinogenesis. Pathology. 2011;43:447.
22. Quiros RM, Ding HG, Gattuso P, et al. Evidence that one subset of anaplastic thyroid carcinomas are derived from papillary carcinomas due to BRAF and p53 mutations. Cancer. 2005;103:2261.
23. Wang H, Huang Y, Huang J, et al. Anaplastic carcinoma of the thyroid arising more often from follicular carcinoma than papillary carcinoma. Ann Surg Oncol. 2007;14:3011.
24. Stoler DL, Nowak NJ, Matsui S, et al. Comparative genomic instabilities of thyroid and colon cancers. Arch Otolaryngol Head Neck Surg. 2007;133:457.
25. Wiseman SM, Griffith OL, Deen S, et al. Identification of molecular markers altered during transformation of differentiated into anaplastic thyroid carcinoma. Arch Surg. 2007;42:717.
26. Schiff BA, McMurphy AB, Jasser SA, et al. Epidermal growth factor receptor (EGFR) is overexpressed in anaplastic thyroid cancer, and the EGFR inhibitor gefitinib inhibits the growth of anaplastic thyroid cancer. Clin Cancer Res. 2004;10:8594.
27. Gule MK, Chen Y, Sano D, et al. Targeted Therapy of VEGFR2 and EGFR significantly inhibits growth of anaplastic thyroid cancer in an orthotopic murine model. Clin Cancer Res. 2011;17:2281.
28. Derbel O, Limem S, Segura-Ferlay C, et al. Results of combined treatment of anaplastic thyroid carcinoma (ATC). BMC Cancer. 2011;11:469.
29. Tennvall J, Lundell G, Wahlberg P, et al. Anaplastic thyroid carcinoma: three protocols combining doxorubicin, hyperfractionated radiotherapy and surgery. Br J Cancer. 2002;86:1848.

30. De Crevoisier R, Baudin E, Bachelot A, et al. Combined treatment of anaplastic thyroid carcinoma with surgery, chemotherapy, and hyperfractionated accelerated external radiotherapy. Int J Radiation Oncology Biol Phys. 2004;60:1137.
31. Foote RL, Molina JR, Kasperbauer JL, et al. Enhanced survival in locoregionally confined anaplastic thyroid carcinoma: a single-institution experience using aggressive multimodal therapy. Thyroid. 2011;21:25.
32. Higashiyama T, Ito Y, Hirokawa M, et al. Optimal surgical procedure for locally curative surgery in patients with anaplastic thyroid carcinoma: importance of preoperative ultrasonography. Endocr J. 2010;57:763.
33. Sugino K, Ito K, Mimura T, et al. The important role of operations in the management of anaplastic thyroid carcinoma. Surgery. 2002;131:245.
34. Lang BH, Lo C. Surgical options in undifferentiated thyroid carcinoma. World J Surg. 2007;31:969.
35. Pierie JEN, Muzikansky A, Randall MA, et al. The effect of surgery and radiotherapy on outcome of anaplastic thyroid carcinoma. Ann Surg Oncol. 2002;9:57.
36. Holting T, Meybier H, Buhr H. Status of tracheotomy in treatment of the respiratory emergency in anaplastic thyroid cancer. Wien Klin Wochenschr. 1990;102:264–6.
37. Bhatia A, Rao A, Ang K, et al. Anaplastic thyroid cancer: clinical outcomes with conformal radiotherapy. Head Neck. 2010;32:829.
38. Troch M, Koperek O, Sheuba C, et al. High efficacy of concomitant treatment of undifferentiated (anaplastic) thyroid cancer with radiation and docetaxel. J Clin Endocrinol Metab. 2010;95:E54.
39. Higashiyama T, Ito Y, Hirokawa M, et al. Induction chemotherapy with weekly paclitaxel administration for anaplastic thyroid carcinoma. Thyroid. 2010;20:7.
40. Kurebayashi J, Okubo S, Yamamoto Y, et al. Additive antitumor effects of gefitinib and imatinib on anaplastic thyroid cancer cells. Cancer Chemother Pharmacol. 2006;58:460.
41. Podtcheko A, Ohtsuro A, Namba H, et al. Inhibition of ABL tyrosine kinase potentiates radiation-induced terminal growth arrest in anaplastic thyroid cancer cells. Radiat Res. 2006;165:35–42.
42. Kim E, Matsuse M, Saenko V, et al. Imatinib enhances docetaxel-induced apoptosis through inhibition of nuclear factor-kB activation in anaplastic thyroid carcinoma cells. Thyroid. 2012;22:717–24.
43. Ha H, Lee J, Urba S, et al. A phase II study of imatinib in patients with advanced anaplastic thyroid cancer. Thyroid. 2010;20:975.
44. Bible K, Suman V, Menefee M, et al. A multi-institutional phase 2 trial of pazopanib monotherapy in advanced anaplastic thyroid cancer. J Clin Endocrinol Metab. 2012;97:1379.
45. Yu X, Phan T, Patel PN, et al. Chrysin activates notch1 signaling and suppresses tumor growth of anaplastic thyroid carcinoma in vitro and in vivo. Cancer. 2013;119:774–81.
46. Lin S, Yu Z, Riedl C, et al. Treatment of anaplastic thyroid carcinoma in vitro with a mutant vaccinia virus. Surgery. 2007;142:976.
47. Alfano RW, Leppla SH, Liu S, et al. Inhibition of tumor angiogenesis by the matrix metalloproteinase-activated anthrax lethal toxin in an orthotopic model of anaplastic thyroid carcinoma. Mol Cancer Ther. 2010;9:190–201.
48. Kojic SL, Strugnell SS, Wiseman SM. Anaplastic thyroid cancer: a comprehensive review of novel therapy. Expert Rev Anticancer Ther. 2011;11:387.

External Beam Radiotherapy for Thyroid Cancer

10

Harvey Quon

Treatment of differentiated thyroid cancer (DTC) most often involves a combination of surgery, radioactive iodine (RAI) and suppression of thyroid-stimulating hormone (TSH). In specific situations, external beam radiotherapy (EBRT) could be of benefit, although this remains controversial because of a lack of randomized evidence to support its use. In contrast, EBRT is of standard use in the multimodal management of anaplastic thyroid cancer (ATC) with surgery and systemic agents. Despite this, outcomes remain poor, supporting the need for additional research of this devastating disease. This chapter focuses on the role of EBRT in DTC and ATC.

Differentiated Thyroid Cancer

Adjuvant EBRT

In some patients, the risk of locoregional recurrence of DTC remains high, despite total thyroidectomy and RAI. This has prompted the use of EBRT in an attempt to improve local control. Most commonly, indications for adjuvant EBRT include extra thyroidal extension and residual tumour, particularly if the disease is non-RAI-avid. Also, given the favourable prognosis of young patients, EBRT is typically reserved for older patients in whom the risk of disease progression is higher.

The clinical evidence supporting the role of adjuvant EBRT in the treatment of DTC has predominantly come from single-institution, retrospective studies, which must be interpreted with caution given the potential for selection bias [1–6]. The

H. Quon
Radiation Oncology, CancerCare Manitoba,
675 McDermot Avenue, Winnipeg, MB R3E 0V9, Canada
e-mail: hquon@cancercare.mb.ca

© K. Alok Pathak, Richard W. Nason, Janice L. Pasieka, Rehan Kazi, Raghav C. Dwivedi 2015
Springer India/Byword Books
K.A. Pathak et al. (eds.), *Management of Thyroid Cancer: Special Considerations*, Head and Neck Cancer Clinics, DOI 10.1007/978-81-322-2434-1_10

Table 10.1 American Thyroid Association (ATA) and British Thyroid Association (BTA) guidelines for adjuvant EBRT in DTC

ATA [8]	Over age of 45 years with grossly visible extrathyroidal extension at the time of surgery and a high likelihood of microscopic residual disease
	Gross residual tumour for whom further surgery or RAI would probably be ineffective
BTA [9]	Gross evidence of local tumour invasion at surgery, presumed to have significant macro-or microscopic residual disease, particularly if the residual tumour fails to concentrate sufficient amounts of RAI
	Extensive pT4 disease in patients >60 years of age, with extensive extranodal spread after optimal surgery, even in the absence of evident residual disease

RAI radioactive iodine, *EBRT* external beam radiotherapy, *DTC* differentiated thyroid cancer

only randomized trial evaluating the role of adjuvant EBRT was closed early on account of poor accrual [7]. However, on the basis of available evidence, the British Thyroid Association (BTA), Royal College of Physicians, and American Thyroid Association (ATA) have published guidelines for the use of EBRT in DTC [8, 9]. A summary of these is listed in Table 10.1.

In a study by Farahati et al., 169 patients with pT4N0-1M0 DTC underwent total thyroidectomy, RAI therapy and TSH suppression between 1979 and 1992 in Germany [1]. Ninety-nine patients underwent adjuvant EBRT to the neck, consisting of 50–60 Gy followed by a 6–10 Gy boost to high-risk regions. The planning target volume included the thyroid bed, anterior neck from mastoid or hyoid down to carina, and the supraclavicular regions. The addition of EBRT improved locoregional recurrences (p=0.004) and distant failures (p=0.0003).

In an analysis of 382 patients with DTC treated at the Princess Margaret Hospital (Canada) between 1958 and 1985, multivariate analysis revealed that age of >60 years, tumour size of >4 cm, multifocality, postoperative residual disease, lymph node involvement, less extensive surgery and lack of use of RAI were significant predictors of locoregional failure [3]. Whereas EBRT was not found to improve locoregional control or cause-specific survival (CSS) in the entire cohort of patients, a beneficial effect was found for the subgroup of 155 patients with papillary histology and microscopic residual disease with 10-year CSS of 100 % vs. 95 % (p=0.038) and 10-year local relapse-free rate of 93 % vs. 78 % (p=0.01) for those with EBRT versus those without, respectively.

More recent reports have also been published examining outcomes of patients treated with EBRT using more modern radiotherapy techniques. In a retrospective analysis from MD Anderson (USA), 131 patients with DTC who received EBRT between 1996 and 2005 were examined [5]. Of these, 96 % had extraglandular disease and 47 % had positive surgical margins. Patients underwent a median 60 Gy using 3-dimensional conformal radiotherapy (3DCRT) or intensity-modulated radiotherapy (IMRT) techniques. With a median follow-up of 38 months, the 4-year locoregional relapse-free survival was 79 %. Multivariate analysis revealed gross residual disease (p<0.0001) and high-risk histological features (Hurthle cell, tall cell, clear cell, or poorly differentiated features) (p=0.0021) predicted for increased risk of locoregional relapse.

At Memorial Sloan-Kettering Cancer Center (USA), 76 patients with non-ATC were treated between 1989 and 2006 [4]. Of these, 84 % had DTC histology and 84 % were T4. Treatment included surgery before EBRT in 93 % and RAI in 74 % of patients. EBRT was delivered with a median of 63 Gy using IMRT in 63 % of patients. The treatment field included 'low-risk' regions, including cervical lymph node regions II–VI and the upper mediastinum. 'High-risk' regions included the thyroid and tumour bed, trachea-oesophageal groove, central nodal compartment and pathologically involved lymph node levels. The 4-year overall locoregional control rate for the entire cohort was 72 %.

Radiotherapy Technique

In relation to the treatment of head and neck cancers (HNCs), IMRT has permitted the development of highly conformal radiotherapy plans, which can sculpt the dose in a concave fashion around important organs at risk, such as the spinal cord, oesophagus, trachea and parotid glands (Fig. 10.1). This was not possible previously by using a 3DCRT technique. Randomized controlled trials have shown that IMRT results in superior salivary gland function and quality of life compared with 2-dimensional and 3DCRT techniques in the treatment of HNCs [10, 11].

Studies examining IMRT specifically for the treatment of thyroid cancer are few. However, many of the benefits seen in the treatment of other HNCs would probably apply. In a radiotherapy planning study, Nutting et al. found that IMRT improved planning target volume coverage and reduced the dose to the spinal cord [12]. This would potentially allow dose escalation or minimization of radiation myelopathy after EBRT. Also, in the previously mentioned study of 131 patients treated with EBRT for DTC from MD Anderson, 56 % underwent 3DCRT and 44 % underwent IMRT [5]. The authors found that IMRT was associated with less frequent severe late radiation toxicity compared with 3DCRT techniques (2 % vs. 12 %, respectively).

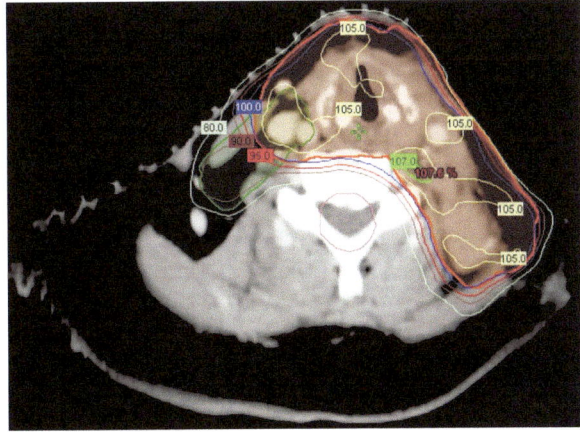

Fig. 10.1 Intensity-modulated radiotherapy plan for thyroid cancer, which shows the ability to generate concave dose distributions that spare organs at risk (e.g. spinal cord)

Radiotherapy Dose and Volume

IMRT is capable of accurately delivering different doses of radiotherapy to separate clinical target volumes (CTVs). The 'high-risk' CTV encompasses gross residual disease and positive margins, the tumour bed, central lymph node region, as well as involved nodal regions. The 'low-risk' CTV includes uninvolved bilateral cervical lymph nodes (levels II–VI) and superior mediastinal lymph node regions. Supporting evidence suggests that treating larger volumes, including the upper mediastinum, might result in improved disease outcomes [13].

In the author's practice, the high-risk CTV volume receives 66 Gy in 33 fractions whereas the low-risk CTV volume receives 59.4 Gy in 33 fractions. Other institutions have also used slightly different dose-fractionation schemes with ≤4 dose-levels, depending on the particular high-risk features involved [5].

Using doses of adjuvant EBRT of >50 Gy is supported by clinical evidence. In one study that examined 41 patients with DTC treated between 1988 and 2001 at two UK cancer centres, indications for EBRT included: (i) macroscopic residual disease (56 %), (ii) microscopic residual disease (24 %), (iii) Hürthle cell variant (7 %), (iv) multiple lymph nodes (7 %), and (v) focus of poor differentiation (5 %) [14]. The target volume was from the mastoid to sternal notch, and laterally the junction of the outer and middle-third of the clavicles. Radiotherapy techniques and doses were variable. Doses ranged from 37.5 to 66 Gy over 3–6.5 weeks, and 35 patients (85 %) received at least one dose of RAI. The 5-year local recurrence rates for patients who received <50 Gy, 50–54 Gy and >54 Gy were 63 %, 15 % and 18 %, respectively (p = 0.02 for trend). The authors concluded that doses of at least 50 Gy were required to improve local control [14].

Toxicity

EBRT for thyroid cancer is associated with acute toxicity, including radiation dermatitis, mucositis, oesophagitis, dysgeusia, dysphagia and laryngitis. Late toxicity can include soft-tissue fibrosis, xerostomia, tracheal stenosis, dysphagia and oesophageal stricture. Also, a second malignancy caused by EBRT is a risk. The use of advanced radiotherapy techniques, such as IMRT, can minimize severe toxicity, as mentioned above.

In the Memorial Sloan-Kettering experience delivering a median 63 Gy, acute grade 3 mucositis was present in 18 % of patients and dysphagia in 32 % [4]. IMRT was used in 63 % of these patients. Late, severe (grade 3+) toxicities were generally rare and present in <5 % of patients (grade 3 xerostomia 1 %, grade 3 dysphagia 4 %, grade 4 laryngeal oedema 2 %) [4]. This rate of late toxicity is comparable to that found in the MD Anderson experience in which patients treated with IMRT had a 2 % incidence of late severe toxicities [5].

Anaplastic Thyroid Cancer

Although rare, ATC often presents with rapid and devastating locoregional symptoms, including dysphagia, dyspnoea, haemoptysis and superior vena cava syndrome [15]. Optimal treatment of ATC involves multimodality therapy with surgery, radiotherapy and systemic agents [16]. The ATA has recently published guidelines for the management of patients with ATC [17].

Outcomes after treatment for ATC remain poor. In a SEER (Surveillance, Epidemiology and End Results) analysis of 516 patients with ATC treated between 1973 and 2000, the overall cause-specific mortality rate was 68.4 % at 6 months and 80.7 % at 12 months [18]. Multivariate analysis revealed that predictors of lower cancer-specific mortality were age of <60 years, intrathyroidal tumour, and the combined use of surgery and EBRT.

Different strategies have been explored to improve outcomes. At the Princess Margaret Hospital, a hyperfractionated radiotherapy regimen has been used for ATC [19]. In a review of 47 patients with ATC who underwent EBRT between 1983 and 2004, 23 underwent radical radiotherapy. Of these 23, 14 underwent once-daily EBRT (60 Gy in 30 fractions over 6 weeks) whereas 9 underwent twice-daily treatment (60 Gy in 40 fractions of 1.5 Gy per fraction twice daily over 4 weeks). The overall local progressionfree rate was 94.1 % at 6 months and 74.1 % at 2 years in this group of patients receiving radical EBRT. Although not statistically significant, the median overall survival in patients with twice-daily EBRT was 13.6 months compared with 10.3 months in the once-daily fractionation group (p = 0.3). No difference was seen in local progression-free survival (p = 0.5). Toxicity of the twice-daily EBRT group was acceptable, with grade 3 acute skin toxicity in 3 patients and no patients with severe oesophageal toxicity. However, other hyperfractionation regimens have been reported with an increased risk of severe toxicities [20, 21].

The addition of chemotherapy continues to be explored. Systemic agents, including doxorubicin and cisplatin, have been used [16, 22]. Recently, there has been interest in the use of taxanes [23–25]. In one study of 6 patients treated with EBRT (60 Gy in 30 fractions) and docetaxel, 4 patients achieved complete remission and 2 experienced a partial response [23]. After 21.5 months of follow-up, 5 patients were alive. However, this regimen was toxic, with hospitalization and severe side-effects in all patients. The integration of novel targeted agents, such as fosbretabulin, imatinib and sorafenib has also been investigated [26–28]. Additional prospective studies with these various agents in conjunction with radiotherapy are needed to further delineate the role for concurrent systemic therapy in the treatment of ATC.

Commentary

K. Alok Pathak

Treatment of differentiated thyroid cancer (DTC) involves surgery with suppression of thyroid-stimulating hormone (TSH), often, in combination with radioactive iodine. The benefit from adjuvant external beam radiotherapy (EBRT) remains controversial in DTC. EBRT has a potential role in older patients with non-iodine-avid residual disease or for extensive pT4 disease with extensive extranodal spread, even in the absence of evident post-surgical residual disease. However, the benefits of EBRT need to be weighed against the acute and longterm toxicities of radiotherapy. EBRT plays a central role in the management of anaplastic thyroid cancer, either alone or in combination with surgery and systemic agents. To enhance the efficacy of radiotherapy, altered fractionation and a combination of radiotherapy and systemic agents have been tried.

Dr Quon has reviewed the available evidence in the literature on the relevance of radiotherapy in the treatment of thyroid cancer, and summarized the guidelines of the British Thyroid Association and American Thyroid Association on the role of EBRT in this disease.

References

1. Farahati J, Reiners C, Stuschke M, et al. Differentiated thyroid cancer. Impact of adjuvant external radiotherapy in patients with perithyroidal tumor infiltration (stage pt4). Cancer. 1996;77:172–80.
2. Tubiana M, Haddad E, Schlumberger M, et al. External radiotherapy in thyroid cancers. Cancer. 1985;55(9 Suppl):2062–71.
3. Tsang RW, Brierley JD, Simpson WJ, et al. The effects of surgery, radioiodine, and external radiation therapy on the clinical outcome of patients with differentiated thyroid carcinoma. Cancer. 1998;82:375–88.
4. Terezakis SA, Lee KS, Ghossein RA, et al. Role of external beam radiotherapy in patients with advanced or recurrent nonanaplastic thyroid cancer: Memorial Sloan-Kettering Cancer Center experience. Int J Radiat Oncol Biol Phys. 2009;73:795–801.
5. Schwartz DL, Lobo MJ, Ang KK, et al. Postoperative external beam radiotherapy for differentiated thyroid cancer: outcomes and morbidity with conformal treatment. Int J Radiat Oncol Biol Phys. 2009;74:1083–91.
6. O'Connell ME, A'Hern RP, Harmer CL. Results of external beam radiotherapy in differentiated thyroid carcinoma: a retrospective study from the Royal Marsden Hospital. Eur J Cancer. 1994;30A:733–9.
7. Biermann M, Pixberg M, Riemann B, et al. Clinical outcomes of adjuvant externalbeam radiotherapy for differentiated thyroid cancer—results after 874 patient-years of follow-up in the MSDS-trial. Nuklearmedizin. 2009;48:89–98; quiz N15.
8. American Thyroid Association (ATA) Guidelines Taskforce on Thyroid Nodules and Differentiated Thyroid Cancer, Cooper DS, Doherty GM, Haugen BR, et al. Revised American Thyroid Association management guidelines for patients with thyroid nodules and differentiated thyroid cancer. Thyroid. 2009;19:1167–214.
9. British Thyroid Association, Royal College of Physicians. Guidelines for the management of thyroid cancer. In: Perros P, editor. Report of the thyroid cancer guidelines update group. 2nd ed. London: Royal College of Physicians; 2007.
10. Nutting CM, Morden JP, Harrington KJ, et al. Parotid-sparing intensity modulated versus conventional radiotherapy in head and neck cancer (parsport): a phase 3 multicentre randomised controlled trial. Lancet Oncology. 2011;12:127–36.
11. Kam MK, Leung SF, Zee B, et al. Prospective randomized study of intensitymodulated radiotherapy on salivary gland function in early-stage nasopharyngeal carcinoma patients. J Clin Oncol. 2007;25:4873–9.

12. Nutting CM, Convery DJ, Cosgrove VP, et al. Improvements in target coverage and reduced spinal cord irradiation using intensity-modulated radiotherapy (IMRT) in patients with carcinoma of the thyroid gland. Radiother Oncol. 2001;60:173–80.
13. Azrif M, Slevin NJ, Sykes AJ, et al. Patterns of relapse following radiotherapy for differentiated thyroid cancer: implication for target volume delineation. Radiother Oncol. 2008;89:105–13.
14. Ford D, Giridharan S, McConkey C, et al. External beam radiotherapy in the management of differentiated thyroid cancer. Clin Oncol (R Coll Radiol). 2003;15:337–41.
15. Smallridge RC, Copland JA. Anaplastic thyroid carcinoma: pathogenesis and emerging therapies. Clin Oncol (R Coll Radiol). 2010;22:486–97.
16. Haigh PI, Ituarte PH, Wu HS, et al. Completely resected anaplastic thyroid carcinoma combined with adjuvant chemotherapy and irradiation is associated with prolonged survival. Cancer. 2001;91:2335–42.
17. Smallridge RC, Ain KB, Asa SL, et al. American Thyroid Association guidelines for management of patients with anaplastic thyroid cancer. Thyroid. 2012;22:1104–39.
18. Kebebew E, Greenspan FS, Clark OH, et al. Anaplastic thyroid carcinoma. Treatment outcome and prognostic factors. Cancer. 2005;103:1330–5.
19. Wang Y, Tsang R, Asa S, et al. Clinical outcome of anaplastic thyroid carcinoma treated with radiotherapy of once- and twice-daily fractionation regimens. Cancer. 2006;107:1786–92.
20. Dandekar P, Harmer C, Barbachano Y, et al. Hyperfractionated accelerated radiotherapy (HART) for anaplastic thyroid carcinoma: toxicity and survival analysis. Int J Radiat Oncol Biol Phys. 2009;74:518–21.
21. De Crevoisier R, Baudin E, Bachelot A, et al. Combined treatment of anaplastic thyroid carcinoma with surgery, chemotherapy, and hyperfractionated accelerated external radiotherapy. Int J Radiat Oncol Biol Phys. 2004;60:1137–43.
22. Swaak-Kragten AT, de Wilt JH, Schmitz PI, et al. Multimodality treatment for anaplastic thyroid carcinoma—treatment outcome in 75 patients. Radiother Oncol. 2009;92:100–4.
23. Troch M, Koperek O, Scheuba C, et al. High efficacy of concomitant treatment of undifferentiated (anaplastic) thyroid cancer with radiation and docetaxel. J Clin Endocrinol Metab. 2010;95:E54–7.
24. Foote RL, Molina JR, Kasperbauer JL, et al. Enhanced survival in locoregionally confined anaplastic thyroid carcinoma: a single-institution experience using aggressive multimodal therapy. Thyroid. 2011;21:25–30.
25. Higashiyama T, Ito Y, Hirokawa M, et al. Induction chemotherapy with weekly paclitaxel administration for anaplastic thyroid carcinoma. Thyroid. 2010;20:7–14.
26. Mooney CJ, Nagaiah G, Fu P, et al. A phase II trial of fosbretabulin in advanced anaplastic thyroid carcinoma and correlation of baseline serum-soluble intracellular adhesion molecule-1 with outcome. Thyroid. 2009;19:233–40.
27. Ha HT, Lee JS, Urba S, et al. A phase II study of imatinib in patients with advanced anaplastic thyroid cancer. Thyroid. 2010;20:975–80.
28. Gupta-Abramson V, Troxel AB, Nellore A, et al. Phase II trial of sorafenib in advanced thyroid cancer. J Clin Oncol. 2008;26:4714–9.

Targeted Therapies in Thyroid Cancer

11

Shabirhusain S. Abadin, Naifa L. Busaidy,
and Nancy D. Perrier

Introduction

Of all thyroid cancers diagnosed yearly worldwide >90 % are considered differentiated thyroid carcinomas (DTC), i.e. papillary or follicular cancers. The majority of patients with these cancers are rendered cured with an operation, radioactive iodine (RAI) ablation, and thyroid-stimulating hormone (TSH) suppression. Therapeutic goals in DTC are first to reduce cancer-specific mortality, second to diminish tumour recurrence, and third to minimize treatment-related morbidity. The mainstay of treatment has been adequate operative resection, typically in the form of a total thyroidectomy with clearance of suspicious or biopsy-positive adenopathy in the lateral and/or central neck compartments. Beyond surgical treatment, RAI and TSH suppression are used as adjuvant therapy for residual or recurrent cancer. Although the patient prognosis is typically good, 5–10 % of patients with an initial diagnosis of thyroid cancer will have tumours that dedifferentiate, resulting in widespread metastatic disease and/or the inability to capture iodine [1]. Most of these patients will succumb to their cancer [1]. For patients with progressive metastatic DTC that is neither surgically resectable nor treated effectively with RAI, treatment options have historically been limited. Cytotoxic chemotherapy with agents, such as doxorubicin, etoposide, taxanes and platinum compounds, has been used to treat patients

S.S. Abadin • N.D. Perrier (✉)
Department of Surgical Oncology, The University of Texas MD Anderson Cancer Center,
1515 Holcombe Blvd., Unit 1484, Houston, TX 77030, USA
e-mail: nperrier@mdanderson.org

N.L. Busaidy
Department of Endocrine Neoplasia and Hormonal Disorders, The University of Texas MD
Anderson Cancer Center, 1515 Holcombe Blvd., Unit 1484, Houston, TX 77030, USA

© K. Alok Pathak, Richard W. Nason, Janice L. Pasieka, Rehan Kazi,
Raghav C. Dwivedi 2015
Springer India/Byword Books
K.A. Pathak et al. (eds.), *Management of Thyroid Cancer: Special Considerations*,
Head and Neck Cancer Clinics, DOI 10.1007/978-81-322-2434-1_11

with aggressive or progressive non-RAI-avid cancer, but such chemotherapy is associated with marginal clinical response rates and toxic side-effects [2].

Medullary thyroid carcinoma (MTC) is diagnosed in approximately 5 % of patients who are diagnosed with thyroid cancer yearly worldwide [3]. Conventional treatment for MTC has been total thyroidectomy and bilateral central neck dissections. RAI and TSH suppression are not used in MTC, as it originates from calcitonin-secreting neuro-endocrine-type cells (parafollicular or C-cells); it is not a follicular-cell derived cancer [3]. Moreover, external beam radiation therapy is used as an adjunct if operative clearance is incomplete. In the setting of distant metastases, therapeutic options have been limited. Indeed, patients with metastatic MTC have poorer outcomes, which are similar to those with radio-resistant DTC. Anaplastic thyroid carcinoma (ATC) has a poor prognosis and management as a rule is palliative.

Over the past decade, molecular events giving rise to thyroid carcinoma have been elucidated, and the relevant signalling pathways have become the targets for new systemic chemotherapeutics. These novel drugs target proteins and elements involved in tumorigenesis and tumour growth or proliferation. Mutant kinases and tumour angiogenesis stimulators are principal targets in this form of intervention. They have been studied in numerous clinical trials but have also been used off-label in selected patients. Although long-term data on disease-free and overall survival is lacking, these agents have provided hope for those patients with progressive thyroid cancer that is not responsive to conventional treatments, namely in terms of limiting the progression of the disease and, in some instances, providing a partial clinical reversal.

Radioactive Iodine (RAI) Ablation

RAI ablation is the earliest form of targeted therapy for DTC. RAI ablation utilizes the physiology of the thyroid gland's propensity for iodine uptake to deliver radioactive-tagged iodine (^{131}I) for destroying follicular-derived thyroid cells via emission of beta rays. This process relies upon iodine uptake in the thyroid and is used to target residual thyroid tissue, persistent DTC, and recurrent DTC. As MTC is not a follicular tumour, RAI ablation is not indicated.

According to the revised American Thyroid Association (ATA) guidelines, postoperative RAI therapy is recommended in patients with persistent disease, namely those with gross residual disease, tumours >4 cm in size in the longest diameter or distant metastatic disease [4]. Furthermore, the recommendations include RAI ablation for those patients with 1–4 cm tumours with lymph node metastases or higher-risk features, including more aggressive histological subtypes (e.g. tall-cell variant), lymphovascular invasion or age >45 years [4]. For patients who have either unifocal or multifocal cancer <1 cm that is confined to the thyroid (i.e. no extrathyroidal extension or invasion to adjacent structures), postoperative RAI ablation is not recommended routinely [4]. When metastatic disease is present and iodine-avid, RAI ablation can be curative in a subset of patients. It is the preferred treatment for recurrent, persistent or metastatic thyroid cancer if a tumour is radio-avid. Complications of RAI ablation are well documented, and in the short term consist of nausea, vomiting, ageusia (loss of taste) and salivary gland swelling. In the long term, sialadenitis is a difficult to treat side-effect. Others include xerostomia, dental caries, pulmonary fibrosis, nasolacrimal duct obstruction, and in the worst case second primary malignancies, including leukaemia or lymphoma [5].

Restoration of RAI Avidity

Return of RAI avidity to non-avid tumours has been seen in laboratory models. Abnormal DNA hypermethylation and histone deacetylation have been implicated in loss of thyroid tumour RAI avidity. Indeed, methylation of the sodium-iodide symporter might play a role in loss of RAI avidity in thyroid cancer [6]. In laboratory models, inhibitors of methylation and histone deacetylation have shown a return of RAI avidity in cell lines, although this has not been seen in clinical application [7]. Romidepsin, a histone deacetylase inhibitor, was studied in one phase I trial and another phase II trial that looked at the Response Evaluation Criteria in Solid Tumours (RECIST) response and the redifferentiation of tumours to an RAI-avid phenotype [8, 9]. Two of 10 patients in the phase II trial showed restoration of RAI uptake. The side-effects of romidepsin can be lethal, with cardiac toxicity as the most serious effect [9].

Traditional Cytotoxic Therapy

Cytotoxic systemic chemotherapy for metastatic thyroid cancers has had limited efficacy. The rates of partial response with multiple agents vary between 25 and 37 % in reported trials [10]. Doxorubicin is the single most effective cytotoxic agent in progressive thyroid cancer; however, it elicits minimal clinical response at the cost of substantial toxicity. This inhibitor of DNA and RNA synthesis is administered intravenously with a recommended bolus dose given every 3 weeks. Its most well-known side-effect is cardiac toxicity, which can result in acute arrhythmias; other toxic effects include leukopenia, infertility and alopecia [2]. One recent report showed that by itself, doxorubicin yielded a partial response (PR) in only 5 % of patients with metastatic thyroid carcinoma at 6 months after treatment [10]. This report did state that patients with lung metastases had a better response than those with bone or nodal disease [10].

Other agents, including etoposide and bleomycin, also show relatively low clinical response rates and considerable toxicity [2].

Other systemic chemotherapies administered in combination with doxorubicin have produced nominal improvements in patient response. One study with doxorubicin, vincristine and bleomycin showed PR in 37.5 % of patients [2]. Generally, response rates with different cytotoxic combinations are rarely complete and the limited PR have typically lasted a few months. Given their toxic profile and low response rates, these traditional cytotoxic therapies are reserved for patients with progressive, symptomatic disease who cannot undergo treatment with the newer targeted agents.

Molecular Basis for Targeted Therapy in Thyroid Cancer

The most recent advance in thyroid cancer treatment is the development of agents that specifically target molecular pathways in thyroid carcinogenesis. To more effectively discuss the variety of agents available either in clinical trials or off-label use, the present authors propose that the following basic schematic of molecular pathways in thyroid cancer is necessary (Fig. 11.1). The mitogen-activated protein kinase (MAPK) pathway in conjunction with interactions with vascular endothelial growth factor receptors (VEGFR) are of utmost importance in tumorigenesis in thyroid cancer. As illustrated in Figure 11.1, in normal cells, cytokines and growth factors activate different types of tyrosine kinase (TK) receptors including RET, which in turn promotes RAS protein phosphorylation. RAS, a membrane-bound G protein, activates RAF, which promotes MAPK and subsequent extracellular signal-regulated kinase phosphorylation and activation. This series of steps leads to proliferative gene expression and subsequent cell growth and proliferation [11]. In thyroid cancer, alterations in RET, RAS and BRAF can give rise to a constitutively active state eliciting tumour initiation and uncontrolled cell growth (Fig. 11.1). The basis for targeted therapy is the inhibition of these oncogenes, in particular the TK

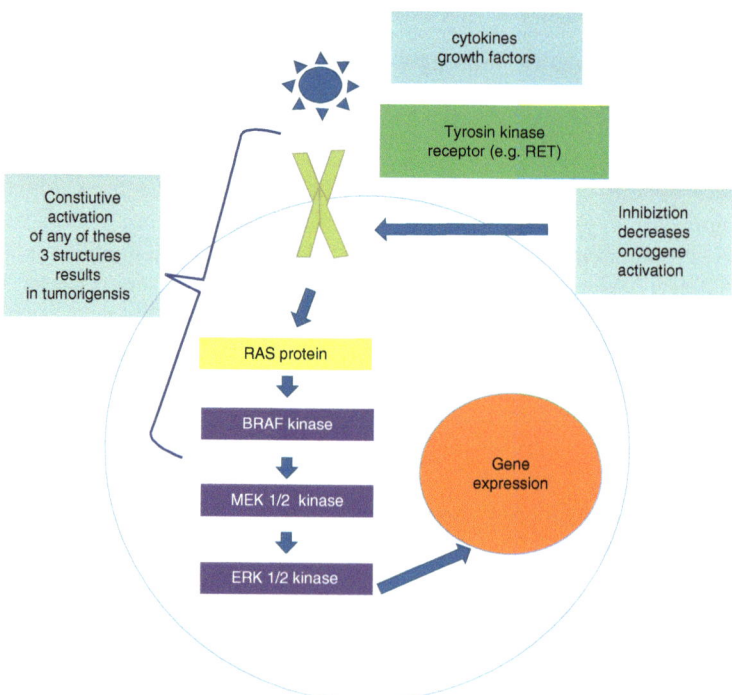

Fig. 11.1 MAPK pathway, TKI receptor inhibition MAPK mitogen-activated protein kinase TK tyrosine kinase

receptor. Approximately 70 % of DTCs arise from single mutations in BRAF, RAS or translocations activating the RET/PTC oncogene [12]. The RET gene encodes for a TK receptor. RET/PTC is produced as a result of chromosomal translocation linking a promoter of the N-terminus of an unrelated gene to the C-terminus of RET, which gives rise to a chimeric protein that is constitutively active in thyroid cancer cells [13]. This mutated protein is a prime initiator of tumour cell growth and has a high prevalence in papillary thyroid cancer (PTC), and is thus labelled the RET/PTC protein [14]. Studies have reported a preponderance of the RET/PTC mutation in microscopic PTC, paediatric DTC and DTC arising after radiation exposure [14]. Given its biology and data for instances in which it predominates, this mutation seems to contribute to tumour initiation and the development of PTC.

Fifty per cent of cases of sporadic MTC result from somatic mutations in the RET gene. The hereditary forms of MTC, including the multiple endocrine neoplasia (MEN) 2A, MEN2B syndromes and familial MTC result from germline mutations in different codons of the RET gene. In MTC, a substitution of a single nucleotide can activate the RET gene, resulting in unencumbered activation of the TK receptor. In familial MTC and MEN2A, the codons commonly mutated are 609, 611, 618 and 620, whereas in MEN2B codon 918 is most common and elicits an especially aggressive clinical pattern. In sporadic MTC, codon 918 is also the most often mutated [3].

Oncogenic activation of BRAF results in more aggressive DTC. The RAF kinase in mammalian cells has three different isoforms—A, B and C. The BRAF kinase isoform is expressed in haematopoietic cells, neurons, testis cells and thyroid follicular cells [14, 15]. The V600E transversion is the most common mutation in BRAF, in which a thymine to adenine transversion occurs at position 1799, resulting in a valine to glutamate substitution at position 600 [14]. The V600E mutation renders BRAF constitutively active. BRAF mutation is the most common genetic change in PTC. Although RET/PTC and RAS mutations are also common, they are independent of each other. Patients with BRAF mutations with PTC have more aggressive properties than PTC without mutations, including a greater likelihood of extrathyroidal invasion and tall-cell variant [16]. Furthermore, normal BRAF produces proteins that aid in follicular cell functions, including the sodium-iodide symporter and the TSH receptor [17]. Thus, when BRAF is mutated, these differentiated functions are diminished. In clinical practice, patients with BRAF mutations have more radio-resistant disease, present with cancers at a more advanced stage, and have a higher incidence of recurrence and mortality [17].

Also targeted in DTC are processes that stimulate tumour growth and development, such as angiogenesis. The VEGFR is activated by other cytokines, hormones and growth factors that stimulate components of MAPK signalling and promote angiogenesis (Fig. 11.2) [17]. Several subtypes of the VEGFR can induce tumour growth and proliferation. With regard to DTC and MTC, the greater the VEGFR expression, the higher the risk of metastasis and recurrence [18].

Inhibitors of VEGFR could act by limiting angiogenesis and the growth of thyroid cancer by restricting the blood supply [18]. These VEGFR inhibitors are thought to stabilize tumour progression more so than preventing tumour initiation.

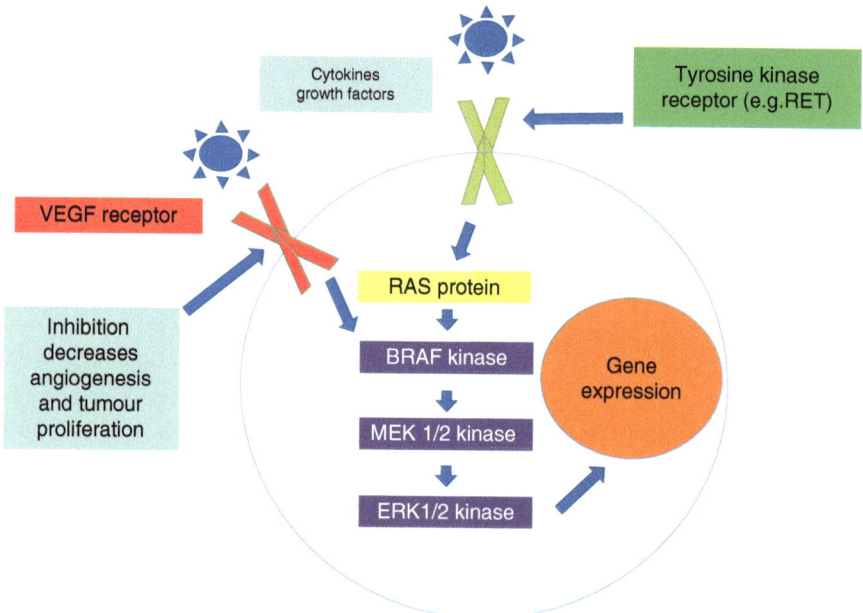

Fig. 11.2 MAPK pathway, VEGF receptor inhibition MAPK mitogen-activated protein kinase VEGF vascular endothelial growth factor

Patient Selection for Targeted Therapy

Determining the proper candidates is critical to optimizing the clinical utility of these novel therapies. In DTC, patients with non-RAI-avid thyroid cancer who are potential candidates for targeted therapy must be comprehensively evaluated on the basis of key clinical factors, including their age and performance status, the extent of disease and the rate of disease progression [19]. Indeed, targeted therapy relies upon patient selection, target identification and specific inhibition of oncogenic cell pathways. In DTC, to be considered for targeted therapy, a patient must have RAI-refractory disease, defined as having at least one lesion without RAI uptake, or those that have progressed within a year after RAI treatment [19]. The overall goal of targeted cancer therapy is to treat tumour cells by using drugs that target the molecular pathways that give rise to tumours, but leave normal cells unaffected. DTC patients have thyroglobulin-positive disease that is non-RAI-avid—meaning the DTC was detected using other imaging modalities. In patients with metastatic thyroid cancer that is relatively stable, based on tumour markers and radiological evaluation, the administration of targeted therapy is questionable, given the relative stability and lower benefit compared with those patients with more aggressive tumour biology. Good candidates for targeted therapy include people pf older age with a poorly differentiated thyroid tumour, with no or low RAI uptake (in DTC), large metastases located in the bones and not lungs, with avid uptake on fludeoxyglucose positron emission tomography (FDG-PET) scan, and rapidly progressive disease [19].

In MTC, patients with distant disease that is progressive and clinically symptomatic should be considered for systemic options, as RAI is not used. Calcitonin and carcinoembryonic antigen (CEA) levels as tumour markers are used to follow these patients, and their doubling times are calculated to determine the rate of progression of their disease. A doubling time of 6 months is thought to be rapid enough to warrant consideration of systemic therapy. Moreover, tumour location in the neck helps guide therapy. For instance, a patient with lateral neck disease that is asymptomatic with progressive distant disease is a reasonable candidate for systemic therapy. In cases of distant metastatic MTC with recurrent or persistent cancer in the central neck, there is concern for initiating systemic therapy, as the risks of doing so include bleeding (near the carotid arteries and jugular veins) and fistula formation (near the trachea or oesophagus). Moreover, patients who are placed on systemic therapies have a higher bleeding risk and consideration of any subsequent operative resection for neck disease will be delayed [20].

Patients with extensive metastatic disease that would potentially cause symptoms are also good candidates for targeted therapy. The speed of progression is evaluated and documented according to the RECIST criteria [21]. Patients with measurable tumours are radiologically monitored using these criteria with radiological testing. Although only a few such patients with thyroid cancer will be candidates for targeted therapy, the clear identification of these patients with reproducible criteria on serial imaging tests is paramount in their selection.

Biologically Targeted Therapies

An understanding of the molecular pathways leading to and promoting thyroid oncogenesis has led to novel systemic therapies, including but not limited to TK inhibitors (TKIs), RET, BRAF and VEGFR inhibitors. Clinical trials should be the first-line therapy for these patients who have systemic, progressive, non-RAI-avid tumours. If a trial is not available or if the patient is not suitable for a trial, off-label use of commercially available targeted therapies should be considered [22]. Available therapies include inhibitors of oncogenic signalling pathways, cell signalling and angiogenesis. TKIs inhibit transmembrane receptors that initiate signalling in the MAPK pathway (Fig. 11.1). TKIs are orally administered and are generally tolerated well [23]. Commercially available TKIs include sorafenib, sunitinib and pazopanib.

Drugs that are not commercially available but are used in clinical trials include motesanib and axitinib. Vemurafenib is a BRAF inhibitor; vandetanib is a RET kinase inhibitor used particularly in MTC [7, 17, 22]. Many of these therapies have inhibitory effects on multiple kinases, including VEGFR inhibition which stabilizes tumour progression (Fig. 11.2). Table 11.1 lists the drugs discussed in this chapter and their molecular targets. Individual side-effects of each drug are discussed, but one that is consistent in many of the therapies is the need to often readjust and

Table 11.1 Targeted therapies for thyroid cancer and their molecular targets

Drug	RET	BRAF	VEGFR	Other
Sorafenib	X	X	2, 3	c-KIT
Sunitinib	X		1, 2, 3	
Motesanib	X		1, 2, 3	c-KIT, PDGFR
Axitinib			1, 2, 3	c-KIT
Pazopanib			1, 2, 3	c-KIT, PDGFR
Vemurafenib		X		
Vandetanib	X		2, 3	RET/PTC3, sporadic/MEN2B RET mutations

VEGF vascular endothelial growth factor

increase thyroid hormone replacement in patients because of malabsorption and/or increased clearance while on targeted therapies. This is especially relevant in those patients with metastatic DTC, as TSH suppression is still an integral part of their treatment.

Sorafenib is a multi-kinase inhibitor of RET, BRAF, and VEGFRs 2 and 3. This drug is approved by the US Food and Drug Administration (FDA) for use only in advanced renal cell carcinoma (RCC) and unresectable hepatocellular carcinoma. Three phase II trials have shown benefit in DTC, with rates of PR of 15–25 % and stable disease (SD) rates at 1 year of 34–61 % [7, 24–27]. A single-institution study showed a clinical benefit of 80 % (20 % PR and 60 % SD) [23]. It further recognized a more pronounced response in lung metastases (22 %) than in nodal disease (0 %) [23]. The median progression-free survival (PFS) was 19 months [23]. As sorafenib has shown benefit in clinical trials, some clinicians have been using this drug as an off-label, non-FDA approved therapy in metastatic non-radioactive-avid thyroid cancer. For MTC, a phase II clinical trial evaluating sorafenib in metastatic MTC showed PR in 1 of 16 patients in the sporadic MTC group, and 14 of the 16 had SD [28]. One patient had PR for 21+ months while 4 patients had SD for ≥15 months. Median PFS was 17.9 months. The initial grouping for the study called for a hereditary arm and a sporadic arm; the hereditary arm was terminated early because of lack of accrual [28]. The side-effects of sorafenib include hand–foot syndrome, rash, fatigue, diarrhoea, QT prolongation, bleeding risks and hypertension. Dermatological changes, including keratoacanthomas and squamous cell carcinoma (SCC) are seen in ≤10 % of patients [25, 29].

Sunitinib is another oral, small molecule TKI that targets VEGFRs 1, 2, 3, and RET. It is FDA-approved for RCC and has been used off-label for metastatic DTC. This drug has shown a PR of 13 % in a phase II trial, with disease stabilization occurring in 68 % of patients, resulting in 81 % clinical benefit [7]. Another phase II study included patients with MTC and DTC and showed a RECIST response on FDG-PET scan in 8 of 29 patients with DTC and 3 of 6 patients with MTC (28 % and 50 %, respectively) [30]. Although the number of patients for MTC was small, a demonstrable decrease of 50 % was also seen in serum calcitonin levels [30]. Side-effects of this drug include fatigue, diarrhoea, palmar or plantar erythrodysesthesia, neutropenia and hypertension [7].

Motesanib is an oral TKI that targets VEGFRs 1, 2, 3, platelet-derived growth factor receptor (PDGFR), c-Kit, and RET. In one phase II study, patients with locally advanced, metastatic or non-radio-avid DTC showed an objective response of 14 % and SD in 67 % [31]. The median PFS was 40 weeks and 81 % patients showed decreased thyroglobulin levels compared to baseline [31]. Another phase II trial showed 81 % SD in a group of patients with progressive, advanced or metastatic MTC [32]. The objective response was low at 2 %. Median PFS was 48 weeks and among tumour marker analysis, an 83 % decrease occurred in serum calcitonin levels. The most common side-effects included diarrhoea, hypertensions and weight loss. Moreover, this drug was especially noted to require an increase in mean dosage of thyroid replacement [32]. Although objective response was low, disease stability was considerable in both studies.

Axitinib is a TKI that selectively inhibits VEGFRs 1, 2, and 3. One phase II trial looking at all histological subtypes (DTC, MTC and ATC) showed PR in 30 % of patients, SD in 38 % of patients, disease progression in 7 % of patients, while 25 % had an indeterminate response or did not undergo post-baseline scans [33]. On tumour assessment using RECIST criteria, of 45 patients with papillary of follicular histology, 14 had PR with a median follow-up of 16.6 months [33]. Nineteen of these 45 patients had SD, 3 had progressive disease, and 9 were deemed indeterminate since they did not meet any response criteria or did not have post-baseline scans [33]. For MTC, 2 of 11 patients had PR and 3 of 11 had SD [33]. Common side-effects of this drug include hypertension, stomatitis, fatigue and diarrhoea [22]. It is important to note that the efficacy of axitinib to induce objective responses and disease stability was in the absence of any anti-RET activity; this suggests that RET may not be as important a target for therapy as VEGFR [7].

Pazopanib is a small-molecule inhibitor of all VEGFR and PDGFR. It is primarily antiangiogenic in its inhibition, with minimal inhibition of RET/PTC or BRAF. In one phase II trial in patients with progressive, metastatic DTC, 32 % showed PR while 6-month PFS was 71 % [34]. The side-effects associated with pazopanib include hypertension (in ≤50 % of patients), liver transaminitis, headache and mucositis. This drug carries a black box warning on account of potential fatal hepatotoxicity [22]. Pazopanib has been recently studied in advanced DTC with hopeful results in vitro. ATC is one of the most deadly human cancers with a median overall survival from diagnosis of 5 months. Historically, taxanes and doxorubicin have been used to palliate patients with advanced ATC; nevertheless, the results are short-lived. In a recent phase II multicentre trial, pazopanib was given to 16 patients, 12 of whom progressed to trial and one suffered death, possibly from treatment-related bleeding [35]. The median survival was 111 days. Although this study had discouraging results with pazopanib as a single agent, perhaps more rational use with combined therapy might offer more benefit in patients with ATC [35].

Vemurafenib is a BRAF mutation inhibitor that has been used in melanoma and colon cancer. Studies on this drug have been limited, as in vitro testing is under way. In a phase I study of vemurafenib on mutated BRAF, 3 of 55 patients had PTC; the remaining 52 had metastatic melanoma [36]. Of the 3 patients, 1 showed PR of lung metastases whereas the other two had prolonged SD [36]. Its side-effects include skin rash, fatigue, pruritus, photosensitivity and nausea [17]. Eleven per cent of patients in this phase I trial had cutaneous SCC [36]. BRAF inhibitors confer a risk of developing cutaneous SCC in ≤5 % of patients [23].

Vandetanib is an oral drug that inhibits RET and VEGFRs 2 and 3. It has been shown to target the RET/PTC 3 mutation, and the M918T RET mutation seen in sporadic MTC and MEN2B [7]. A phase II trial in studying hereditary MTC showed a PR of 20 % with SD of >24 weeks in 73 % of patients [37]. A more recent multi-institutional phase II trial looking at locally advanced or metastatic MTC (both hereditary and sporadic MTC) showed an extrapolated median PFS of 30 months compared with 19 months for placebo [38]. Furthermore, 37 % of patients had progressed and 15 % died during the analysis. The most commonly reported side-effects are rash, diarrhoea, fatigue and QT prolongation [7].

Conclusions

The success of drugs such as all-trans-retinoic acid for acute promyelocytic leukaemia and imatinib mesylate for chronic myelogenous leukaemia illustrates that targeted therapies can work. Nevertheless, the complexities and interplay of multiple cellular pathways and kinases in thyroid cancer teaches us that overcoming drug resistance will be a challenge, and more creative drug regimens and combinations will be necessary to improve patient outcomes.

For thyroid cancer, the rare report of complete responses and the emergence of eventual progression in all of the various monotherapy trials identify the need to develop either more effective single agents or rational combinations of therapeutic targets that have synergistic effectiveness without enhanced cross-toxicities. For this reason, targeting one mutation or oncoprotein may not be sufficient and optimal treatment will probably require combination therapy. Personalized oncology is built on the premise that each person's cancer is unique—with a different aetiology at the molecular level. Clinical guidelines allow for direction in management of patients but do not take into account the nuances and genetic heterozygosities that vary from person to person. These are the very differences that are the foundation of targeted therapy, such as kinase inhibitors.

Another question is why these targeted therapies are not more successful. One reason may be that kinase resistance develops to these drugs [39]. Oncogenic processes may be able to bypass these kinase inhibitors and continue to maintain tumour cell functions and proliferation. In general, these medications show some improvement in reducing tumour volume, but their real benefit is in suppressing progression. In essence, these therapies are more cytostatic than cytotoxic in their tumour response.

Thankfully, most patients diagnosed and treated for thyroid cancer do not warrant treatment with these novel targeted therapies. Nevertheless, a subset population of patients with thyroid cancer progress in their disease state with conventional methods of treatment. For many years, these patients had no good alternative option. Although no pharmacotherapy has shown any benefit in overall or disease-free survival in thyroid cancer, the benefits of PR and disease stabilization provide our patients hope that the rational use of systemic therapy will eventually cure their aggressive cancer.

Commentary

Richard W. Nason

The majority of patients with well-differentiated thyroid cancer (WDTC) have a good prognosis. Medullary thyroid cancer (MTC) is associated with reasonably long survival. These outcomes are achieved with surgery and adjunctive radioactive iodine (RAI) and thyroid-stimulating hormone (TSH) suppression in the former, and surgery alone in the latter.

A small number of patients with progressive local disease and/or distant metastases are not amenable to further standard treatment. Presently, the treatment of these patients is based on historical reports on the response of relatively small cohorts of patients to traditional cytotoxic regimens. The authors of this chapter note that the response rates for these patients are nominal. They comment on the concept of personalized oncology, built on the premise that each person's cancer is unique—with a different aetiology at the molecular level. They cite the success of targeted therapies for select haematological malignancies. The future will see treatment of thyroid cancer tailored to the individual tumour's genetic, epigenetic and proteomic characteristics. Clinicians need to actively support research in this domain.

The use of targeted treatment regimens for thyroid cancer at present requires careful patient selection. The majority of patients with metastatic thyroid cancer in my practice have relatively stable disease and a reasonably good quality of life. Patients selected for these treatments should demonstrate progressive disease that is, or will imminently, become symptomatic.

References

1. Antonelli A, Fallahi P, Ferrari SM, et al. Dedifferentiated thyroid cancer: a therapeutic challenge. Biomed Pharmacother. 2008;62:559–63.
2. Sherman SI. Cytotoxic chemotherapy for differentiated thyroid carcinoma. Clin Oncol (R Coll Radiol). 2010;22:464–8.
3. Hoff AO, Hoff PM. Medullary thyroid carcinoma. Hematol Oncol Clin North Am. 2007;21:475–88.
4. Cooper DS, Doherty GM, Haugen BR, et al. Revised American Thyroid Association management guidelines for patients with thyroid nodules and differentiated thyroid cancer. Thyroid. 2009;19:1167–214.
5. Lee SL. Complications of radioactive iodine treatment of thyroid carcinoma. J Natl Compr Canc Netw. 2010;8:1277–86. quiz 1287.
6. Haugen BR. Redifferentiation therapy in advanced thyroid cancer. Curr Drug Targets Immune Endocr Metabol Disord. 2004;4:175–80.
7. Sherman SI. Targeted therapy of thyroid cancer. Biochem Pharmacol. 2010;80:592–601.

8. Amiri-Kordestani L, Luchenko V, Peer CJ, et al. Phase I trial of a new schedule of romidepsin in patients with advanced cancers. Clin Cancer Res. 2013;19:4499–507.

9. Piekarz RL, Frye R, Turner M, et al. Phase II multi-institutional trial of the histone deacetylase inhibitor romidepsin as monotherapy for patients with cutaneous T-cell lymphoma. J Clin Oncol. 2009;27:5410–7.

10. Matuszczyk A, Petersenn S, Bockisch A, et al. Chemotherapy with doxorubicin in progressive medullary and thyroid carcinoma of the follicular epithelium. Horm Metab Res. 2008;40:210–3.

11. Xing M. BRAF mutation in papillary thyroid cancer: pathogenic role, molecular bases, and clinical implications. Endocr Rev. 2007;28:742–62.

12. Licitra L, Locati LD, Greco A, et al. Multikinase inhibitors in thyroid cancer. Eur J Cancer. 2010;46:1012–8.

13. Santoro M, Melillo RM, Carlomagno F, et al. Molecular mechanisms of RET activation in human cancer. Ann N Y Acad Sci. 2002;963:116–21.

14. Fagin JA. How thyroid tumors start and why it matters: kinase mutants as targets for solid cancer pharmacotherapy. J Endocrinol. 2004;183:249–56.

15. Daum G, Eisenmann-Tappe I, Fries HW, et al. The ins and outs of Raf kinases. Trends Biochem Sci. 1994;19:474–80.

16. Nikiforova MN, Kimura ET, Gandhi M, et al. BRAF mutations in thyroid tumors are restricted to papillary carcinomas and anaplastic or poorly differentiated carcinomas arising from papillary carcinomas. J Clin Endocrinol Metab. 2003;88:5399–404.

17. Sherman SI. Targeted therapies for thyroid tumors. Mod Pathol. 2011;24 Suppl 2:S44–52.

18. Klein M, Vignaud JM, Hennequin V, et al. Increased expression of the vascular endothelial growth factor is a pejorative prognosis marker in papillary thyroid carcinoma. J Clin Endocrinol Metab. 2001;86:656–8.

19. Schlumberger M, Sherman SI. Clinical trials for progressive differentiated thyroid cancer: patient selection, study design, and recent advances. Thyroid. 2009;19:1393–400.

20. You YN, Lakhani V, Wells Jr SA, et al. Medullary thyroid cancer. Surg Oncol Clin N Am. 2006;15:639–60.

21. Therasse P, Arbuck SG, Eisenhauer EA, et al. New guidelines to evaluate the response to treatment in solid tumors. European Organization for Research and Treatment of Cancer, National Cancer Institute of the United States, National Cancer Institute of Canada. J Natl Cancer Inst. 2000;92:205–16.

22. Busaidy NL, Cabanillas ME. Differentiated thyroid cancer: management of patients with radioiodine nonresponsive disease. J Thyroid Res. 2012;2012:618985.

23. Cabanillas ME, Waguespack SG, Bronstein Y, et al. Treatment with tyrosine kinase inhibitors for patients with differentiated thyroid cancer: the MD Anderson experience. J Clin Endocrinol Metab. 2010;95:2588–95.

24. Kloos R, Ringer M, Knopp M, et al. Significant clinical and biologic activity of RAF/VEGF-R kinase inhibitor BAY 43-9006 in patients with metastatic papillary thyroid carcinoma (PTC): updated results of a phase II study. J Clin Oncol. 2006;24:5534.

25. Gupta-Abramson V, Troxel AB, Nellore A, et al. Phase II trial of sorafenib in advanced thyroid cancer. J Clin Oncol. 2008;26:4714–9.

26. Brose MS, Troxel AB, Redlinger M, et al. Effect of BRAFV600E on response to sorafenib in advanced thyroid cancer patients. J Clin Oncol. 2009;27:6002.

27. Hoftijzer H, Heemstra KA, Morreau H, et al. Beneficial effects of sorafenib on tumor progression, but no on radioiodine uptake, in patients with differentiated thyroid carcinoma. Eur J Endocrinol. 2009;161:923–31.

28. Lam ET, Ringel MD, Kloos RT, et al. Phase II clinical trial of sorafenib in metastatic medullary thyroid cancer. J Clin Oncol. 2010;28:2323–30.

29. Kloos RT, Ringel MD, Knopp MV, et al. Phase II trial of sorafenib in metastatic thyroid cancer. J Clin Oncol. 2009;27:1675–84.

30. Carr LL, Mankoff DA, Goulart BH, et al. Phase II study of daily sunitinib in FDG-PET-positive, iodine-refractory differentiated thyroid cancer and metastatic medullary carcinoma of the thyroid with functional imaging correlation. Clin Cancer Res. 2010;16:5260–8.

31. Sherman SI, Wirth LJ, Droz JP, et al. Motesanib diphosphate in progressive differentiated thyroid cancer. N Engl J Med. 2008;359:31–42.

32. Schlumberger MJ, Elisei R, Bastholt L, et al. Phase II study of safety and efficacy of motesanib in patients with progressive or symptomatic, advanced or metastatic medullary thyroid cancer. J Clin Oncol. 2009;27:3794–801.

33. Cohen EE, Rosen LS, Vokes EE, et al. Axitinib is an active treatment for all histologic subtypes of advanced thyroid cancer: results from a phase II study. J Clin Oncol. 2008;26:4708–13.

34. Bible KC, Suman VJ, Molina JR, et al. Efficacy of pazopanib in progressive, radioiodine-refractory, metastatic differentiated thyroid cancers: results of a phase 2 consortium study. Lancet Oncol. 2010;11:962–72.

35. Bible KC, Suman VJ, Menefee ME, et al. A multi-institutional phase 2 trial of pazopanib monotherapy in advanced anaplastic thyroid cancer. J Clin Endocrinol Metab. 2012;97:3179–84.

36. Flaherty KT, Puzanov I, Kim KB, et al. Inhibition of mutated, activated BRAF in metastatic melanoma. N Engl J Med. 2010;363:809–19.

37. Wells Jr SA, Gosnell JE, Gagel RF, et al. Vandetanib for the treatment of patients with locally advanced or metastatic hereditary medullary thyroid cancer. J Clin Oncol. 2010;28:767–72.

38. Wells Jr SA, Robinson BG, Gagel RF, et al. Vandetanib in patients with locally advanced or metastatic medullary thyroid cancer: a randomized, double-blind phase III trial. J Clin Oncol. 2012;30:134–41.

39. Loges S, Mazzone M, Hohensinner P, et al. Silencing or fueling metastasis with VEGF inhibitors: antiangiogenesis revisited. Cancer Cell. 2009;15:167–70.